FED UP!

FED UP!

Winning the War Against Childhood Obesity

Susan Okie, M.D.

Joseph Henry Press
Washington, D.C.

Joseph Henry Press   500 Fifth Street, NW   Washington, D.C. 20001

The Joseph Henry Press, an imprint of the National Academies Press, was created with the goal of making books on science, technology, and health more widely available to professionals and the public. Joseph Henry was one of the founders of the National Academy of Sciences and a leader in early American science.

Library of Congress Cataloging-in-Publication Data
Okie, Susan.
  Fed up! : winning the war against childhood obesity / Susan Okie.
      p. ; cm.
  Includes bibliographical references and index.
  ISBN 0-309-09310-4 (hardcover)
  1. Obesity in children—United States. 2. Obesity in children—United States—
Prevention.
  [DNLM: 1. Obesity—epidemiology—United States—Popular Works. 2. Obe-
sity—prevention & control—United States—Popular Works. WD 212 O41f 2005]
  I. Title: Winning the war against childhood obesity. II. Title.
  RJ399.C6O383 2005
  618.92′398—dc22
                          2004026618

Printed in the United States of America.

To Meagan, Bruce, Adam, Trianna, Brian, and the other girls and boys who shared a difficult part of their lives with me; and to my family—Walter, Pete, and Jake.

Contents

Foreword

The childhood obesity epidemic poses a major threat to our nation's future adults. *Fed Up!* comes none too soon as a guide to bringing this public health emergency under control. We have become one of the world's fattest nations. No previous U.S. generation has raised children likely to have a shorter life expectancy than their parents. But we are not powerless to prevent obesity in our children. Dr. Okie's book alerts parents to the dangers *and* the solutions. It does take a village to raise a child, so parents who want to provide their children with a healthy future will need to join together and fight for it from earliest childhood on.

Since obesity can be identified in early childhood and is easier to prevent than to treat, it should be a focus in every pediatric well-child care visit. Not all overweight children will become obese adults, but they are at greater risk. Obesity in childhood threatens our children's future, increasing their risk for high blood pressure and heart disease, strokes, diabetes, lung problems, arthritis, and other musculoskeletal disorders. The potential for psychological damage to an obese child who faces teasing and rejection should also be in every parent's mind. As the obesity epidemic captures the headlines, the stigmatization is only likely to intensify. Dr. Okie sensitively addresses this issue while pointing out that avoiding a child's weight problem altogether will not protect his or her self esteem.

Obesity does not strike all equally. The tendency toward obesity is inherited, though poor nutrition and inadequate physical activity play an important role in turning this vulnerability into a reality. In the United States, Mexican American, African American, and Native American children are more likely to be obese than non-Hispanic white children. While genetics may play a role in some cases, higher rates of poverty and cultural values are embedded in these discrepancies. In certain cultures where poverty is associated with a food scarcity, parents may feel pride in providing their children with foods touted on TV. They may also value a well-padded child as one who is safe from the malnutrition that earlier generations have experienced or from violence on the street where the child lives. Poverty is a powerful factor, because healthy foods are more expensive and more difficult to find in poor neighborhoods.

Kelly Brownell, director of the Yale Center for Eating and Weight Disorders, calls our communities "toxic environments." Our attitudes toward exercise are reflected in schools that are cutting out recess and physical education classes. Achievement test results are now the key to funding and have become the sole focus at many public schools. Too often children's need for time to move about and play in order to learn is ignored. In many communities playgrounds and neighborhoods are no longer safe places for children to play and learn sports. As a result children invest most of their after-school time in passive activities with television and video games and so fail to get the exercise they need. The hours of television they watch correlates with the unhealthy, excess weight that they accumulate.

Marketing aimed directly at children and bypassing parents can also be toxic. Television programming for children is saturated with junk food ads. Marketers know that it pays off to disempower parents and push children to beg for the most aggressively advertised foods. The sweetest, saltiest, and fattiest products are the cheapest to manufacture and the most likely to exert an addictive pull—especially on young, inexperienced taste buds. Most working parents have limited time with their children and must compete with the marketers for their hearts and minds. They are forced to struggle against the tempting misinformation of advertisements and resist their children's demands for cereals or soft drinks or fast food "just like the ones on TV." Psychologist Susan Linn has recommended a "commercial-free childhood" to protect our children from the toxic effects of the media around them.

Fed Up! is a hopeful book that shows how the battle against obesity can be won. As parents we must begin to fight for a healthy environment for our children. We need to stand up and voice our demands. Our communities need to stand together for a healthy future *for all children.*

As Dr. Okie's book so clearly demonstrates, the occurrence of the obesity epidemic at the beginning of the twenty-first century, and its spread from the epicenter in the United States to countries with similar economies is no accident. It is rooted in the changed relationships of humans to sources of sustenance and to physical activities required for survival. The majority of our population no longer has a direct role in food production. For most, physical work to obtain food is no longer necessary and knowledge about food—what to grow and what is necessary for survival and health—is no longer handed down through the experience of one generation to the next. Instead, we eat our food—fast food, take-out food, catered food, frozen food, microwaveable food—without expending significant calories to obtain it. The kinds of foods that are available are dictated by marketing and profit margins. Our obesity crisis is unfolding in societies, like ours, that redirect human activity away from calorie expenditure and food consumption away from satisfying caloric and nutritional necessity.

The fight for affordable, healthy foods; safe opportunities for physical activity; and freedom from toxic marketing goes beyond what any one parent or family can accomplish alone. Together we must advocate for the following:

• *Opportunities for physical activity*—funding for daily physical education programs with qualified instructors and safe equipment in public schools; safe parks; neighborhoods suited for outdoor play such as walking, running, biking, and other sports; and community planning that allows inhabitants to safely walk rather than drive to school, work, and stores.

• *Access to healthy food and protection against unhealthy food—*

affordable fresh produce, grains, dairy products, fish, poultry, and meats must be available in local stores in every community, rich or poor. Huge megastores on the outskirts of towns have supplanted smaller shops in the town centers so that residents must drive rather than walk. Once there they'll be more likely to buy longer-lasting processed foods in packages and cans (so they won't need to return as often) that often contain higher levels of salt, unhealthy fats, and simple carbohydrates. In poor communities, cheaper processed foods are often all that are available on the shelves of local stores. School meals must be nutritionally sound. Limiting children's access to unhealthy foods—as is done for alcohol and cigarettes—is also essential (for example, removing soda and candy machines from schools).

• *An end to nutritional misinformation*—food marketing found on television, radio, magazines, billboards, the Internet, and food packaging floods consumers with misinformation and deceptively positive associations to unhealthy foods, drowning out the effects of accurate information that is far less available. Children are especially vulnerable, yet are specifically targeted. Advertising for cigarettes, a public health hazard, was sharply curtailed several decades ago. It is time to do the same thing for nutritionally empty foods.

Without these changes we will lose this struggle. Alone, our power as parents will not suffice. We must work together for new political and economic priorities that put a healthy future for our children first. Dr. Okie's important book is a battle cry, one that can lead us all to community action that will save generations to come from the threat of obesity.

T. Berry Brazelton, M.D.
Joshua Sparrow, M.D.
Children's Hospital
Boston, Massachusetts

Author's Note

I wrote this book in the hope of empowering parents and others to respond to an epidemic that threatens children's health. My own painful memories of being an overweight child provided emotional fuel for the project. I also brought to it my prevention-oriented training as a family physician, my many years of experience as a medical reporter for the *Washington Post*, and the lessons that I have learned as the mother of two boys.

To understand what might be causing an epidemic of childhood obesity, it is important for readers to gain a fundamental understanding of three key areas related to the crisis: how the human body regulates appetite and maintains itself at a constant weight; how the genes that children inherit from their parents contribute to their chances of becoming overweight; and how some environmental changes in the past 30 to 40 years may be interfering with our bodies' ability to maintain a healthy weight, making more and more of us, young and old, store too much fat tissue. I provide readers with the information to develop a working knowledge of these areas with the help of researchers, specialists who treat overweight children, and other professionals from various disciplines who have shared their insights, discoveries, and concerns. I also describe the scientific evidence supporting assorted changes in diet or lifestyle as effective strategies for slowing or halting the rise in obesity among kids.

There is probably no single cause or simple solution to this obesity epidemic. Many factors are likely contributing, and we don't yet know which are paramount. But parents and other adults are certainly not powerless. Researchers have already identified steps that can be taken at home, at school, and in the community to reduce a child's risk of becoming overweight. There is much that we can do. This book offers the tools.

In researching *Fed Up!* I spent time with many children in a variety of settings. I talked with them, observed them in classrooms, ate lunch with them in school cafeterias, hung out with them on playgrounds, gardened and cooked with them, and accompanied them on visits to dietitians and clinics. All of the children, teenagers, and adults described are real individuals. No one is fictitious or a composite. I have referred to the kids and their parents by first names only to protect their privacy.

Many people helped me on this project, and I have tried to thank them all in a separate acknowledgments section. Above all, I am grateful to the children and families who let me into their lives and allowed me to write about their own struggles with obesity in order to help other kids.

CHAPTER 1

The Fattest Generation

Meagan gets up early, before her father and brother are awake, and fries up a batch of soy bacon. Ten and a half years old, she is a committed vegetarian who likes the taste of meat, and she is ravenous. She washes the bacon down with a glass of water, then gets ready for school. She's in the fifth grade at a public school about 2 miles from her home in Palos Verdes, a seaside Los Angeles suburb. Meagan has shiny brown hair in a ponytail and new glasses. Smart and funny, she's an extrovert who loves to sing and dance and to tend goal in soccer games. Recently, though, she has gained a lot of weight, especially around her middle—a fact that has started to provoke occasional teasing by classmates and to worry her parents, both of them doctors who have been treating heart disease, high blood pressure, and other complications of obesity in adults for their entire careers.

Meagan has seen a dietitian, who taught her about portion sizes and how to rate her hunger on a scale of 1 to 10. She would like to be leaner, to put a stop to the teasing, and to be able to move faster in soccer, but she also wants to be in charge of her own life and of what she eats. She loves sweets and can name all the doughnut and ice cream stores near her neighborhood. She's especially partial to one ice cream parlor where you can choose your favorite candy bar or chocolate chips and they "mush it in."

This morning traffic is bumper to bumper on the way to school. Although there's a bike lane beside the road, Meagan rarely rides to school. Despite their concerns about the traffic, her parents have been urging her to do so for the sake of the exercise, but she has difficulty pedaling the steepest part of the route, and she can't transport her cornet by bicycle on band practice days. Driving her to school is usually easier for her mother and father than overcoming her resistance.

The elementary school is a cluster of single-story buildings connected by courtyards and walkways, backed by playgrounds and a large grassy field for soccer and other games. After the first bell rings, students are allowed a few minutes on the playground. Meagan waits for a turn to spin on a big tire swing. Ten minutes and one spin later, the second bell sends her off to homeroom.

This morning Meagan and her best friend, Julia, are assigned a special activity: they are to research bridge design on the Internet and build an example using dried pasta and glue. Hoping to make an arch, they painstakingly glue tubes of macaroni end to end, but their constructions keep falling apart. Eventually they settle for laying out noodles side by side to make a beam bridge. Ninety minutes go by, and the girls get hungry. They munch on pieces of dried spaghetti.

At recess the two go outside to the courtyard. Julia, chatty, slender, and constantly in motion, unscrews a thermos of steaming hot chocolate and opens a plastic bag of marshmallows.

"Meagan, you want hot chocolate?"

"Mmm, tasty," says Meagan, slurping a cupful. "Maybe we can dip the noodles."

Friends join them and Julia passes around the marshmallows. The girls throw them in the air and catch them in their mouths. They compete to see who can do the highest cancan kicks, then the widest split. "I'm going to break my jeans if I do a split," Meagan predicts. Instead, she breaks into a spirited rendition of "Freedom Bound," a song from the fifth-grade play, and the others join in. The girls end recess on a high note, dancing and shouting out the song.

Back in homeroom, Meagan's teacher, Lydia Day, assigns a writing exercise, then conducts a poetry lesson. At 12:30 the bell rings for lunch.

The day's main offering in the school cafeteria is a chicken leg served with barbecue sauce or ketchup. Meagan decides on the vegetarian alternative, a bean and cheese burrito. Both entrees come with hash brown potatoes, a large roll, and a strawberry ice, and students are free to complete their lunch with celery, apples, orange slices, or wilted-looking lettuce from a salad table. Meagan grabs some celery sticks and a carton of chocolate milk. She and five friends squeeze onto benches around a table. Julia passes around tortilla chips, salsa, marshmallows, and hot chocolate, collecting in return four strawberry ices. Meagan eats her burrito and hash browns, some celery and chips, and then goes back to the cafeteria to buy an ice cream bar. By the time everyone's finished eating only five minutes of lunch period remain. Meagan and two friends head quickly for the playground and a brief tug-of-war over who will get to play with a tetherball suspended from a pole. The bell rings.

Back in class, Meagan and her schoolmates read aloud from a children's novel, *Mrs. Frisby and the Rats of NIMH*, and write answers to questions on a worksheet. At 2:15 the bell rings for the twice-weekly physical education class.

"Three laps," barks a P.E. teacher as about 100 fifth-graders spill out onto the soccer field. The kids start running around the perimeter; Meagan and her friends slow to a walk on the far side, then begin jogging as they approach the teachers. They finish their laps and a game of capture-the-flag, a chaotic form of mass tag, gets under way. The goal is to run past enemy team members without being tagged, get inside a hula hoop marking a safe zone, and capture a Frisbee. Anyone tagged goes to "jail" and waits by one of the soccer goals to be liberated. At any moment dozens of people are running in all directions while dozens of others are standing in safe territory or waiting in jail. Periodically Ms. Day yells "Jail break!" and the prisoners rush back onto the field. Meagan at one point successfully evades opposing team members and makes it all the way to the hula hoop but can't capture the Frisbee. When the bell rings at 3:15 she lingers for a few minutes to talk to friends before heading home.

Meagan's street, a quiet cul-de-sac, looks deserted. Since her parents are still at work, she gets a canned juice drink from the pantry and lounges on their bed with a favorite magazine. At length, recalling that her science project is due the next day, she begins her homework. Most of Meagan's afternoons are spent like this. She'd like to play soccer instead, but the sport is available only through after-school leagues, and girls in her age group must compete for spots. She tried out for a select team, but wasn't chosen. There isn't a noncompetitive soccer league for girls in the area, so for now she has no opportunity to play the game.

Meagan's brother comes home from middle school, and her father returns from his office at a local hospital. Her dad gets out the fish that's been marinating in the refrigerator and broils it while boiling potatoes and steaming string beans. Meagan eats a banana and requests meatless chicken noodle soup and orange juice for dinner, along with the vegetables; she doesn't eat fish. When her mother arrives, the family sits down to eat. Finishing before her parents do, she entertains them by belting out her version of "Freedom Bound"—singing all the parts, dancing in the style of Britney Spears, and laughing uproariously. It's the most vigorous exercise she's gotten all day.

🐾🐾🐾

Compared with many kids in the United States, Meagan is lucky: she has well-educated and successful parents, she has a pantry stocked with nutritious foods, and she attends a good public school in one of the most health-conscious districts in the nation. At 10 she already knows more about the importance of good eating and exercise habits than many adults, yet like many other American kids, she is struggling with a problem that is causing her emotional distress and that may imperil her future health, a problem that poses an unprecedented threat to millions of children. She is overweight.

Throughout human history, until the end of the twentieth century, the vast majority of the world's children have been lean. Now, all of a sudden, at beaches, playgrounds, and amusement parks, over-weight children—as well as overweight adults—are numerous and conspicuous. In the past 30 years rates of child obesity in the United States and in many other countries have soared, and diseases caused by excess weight are correspondingly on the rise, even in the very young.

As Americans, many of us have become resigned to hearing that we are citizens of one of the world's fattest nations. Almost two-thirds of U.S. adults are overweight or obese, according to standardized defi-nitions based on the links between excess body-fat stores and the risk of disease. We regularly read depressing new statistics about our na-tional weight problem or listen to warnings from doctors about its likely future effect on our collective health. We feel guilty. We vow to eat less or to exercise more. Sometimes we act on those resolutions; perhaps more often we end up feeling defeated by the difficulty of mak-ing lasting changes in our habits.

But we cannot afford to remain helpless or resigned in the face of what is now happening to children and adolescents in our own coun-try and in much of the rest of the world, including Latin America, Canada, Europe, the Middle East, Australia, Japan, India, and China. Since the 1970s the prevalence of obesity in the United States has more than tripled among children aged 6 to 11 and has more than doubled among children aged 2 to 5 and adolescents between 12 and 19. An estimated nine million boys and girls over the age of 6, representing about 15 percent of the nation's children, are currently obese. An ap-proximately equal number weigh more than is desirable for their health and are considered "at risk" of becoming obese. The epidemic has spread to preschool-age children, even toddlers. No group is spared: children of all races, ethnicities, and socioeconomic strata are experi-encing rising rates of obesity, although African Americans, Hispanic Americans, and American Indians are among those most affected.

This unprecedented increase in childhood obesity is a true public health emergency. For many of today's children it signals future health consequences that are likely to be far worse than those suffered by pre-vious generations who became overweight only in adulthood. About half of obese elementary school–age children and about three-quar-ters of obese adolescents grow up to become obese adults who will

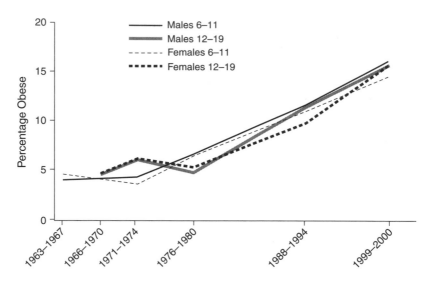

Trends in childhood obesity in U.S. girls and boys aged 6 through 19 years. Obesity is defined as a BMI at or above age- and gender-specific 95th percentile cutoff points taken from the 2000 CDC BMI charts.
Source: See Notes.

likely carry the burden of unhealthy fat throughout their lives, since obesity in adulthood is extremely difficult to overcome. They may become sick in their prime with diseases once associated with old age. And for many children, the medical, emotional, and social consequences of being overweight are already happening. Obese children are often teased, bullied, or ostracized by other kids and may react by losing self-confidence and becoming socially isolated, depressed, or even aggressive. Their bodies, too, are affected: a majority of overweight kids and teenagers have already developed at least one additional risk factor for heart disease, and one-quarter of them have two or more. Unprecedented numbers of U.S. children are being diagnosed with an obesity-related type of diabetes that until recently was called "adult-onset" diabetes.

Indeed, it is time to recognize obesity as a disease in its own right. Even in an otherwise healthy child, excess fat can subtly alter normal metabolic processes and may, over time, damage or disrupt the function of many of the body's organs and systems. In adulthood, people who remain seriously overweight have elevated rates of heart disease, diabetes, high blood pressure, high cholesterol, breathing disorders, cancer, liver and gallbladder disease, arthritis, and depression. Many of these complications of obesity are increasingly showing up in children and teenagers.

The growing numbers of obese children in the United States and in many other countries are victims of an epidemic just as surely as if they were infected with a virus. We tend to think of an epidemic as an outbreak of a contagious illness. But to public health scientists the sudden upswing in obesity rates that occurred at the end of the twentieth century is every bit as dramatic and unexpected as an outbreak of a new infectious disease and has begun to trigger the kind of alarm that might greet the global resurgence of polio. In the fall of 2003, Julie Gerberding, the director of the federal Centers for Disease Control and Prevention (CDC), the government agency best known for fighting infectious diseases and bioterrorism, declared obesity the number one health threat facing the United States.

🐜🐜🐜

The seventh-graders in Christine Mattis's health class at D. W. Griffith Junior High, in East Los Angeles, have not heard the words "obesity" and "epidemic" before. Most of them come from Mexican American families, a population with especially high obesity rates. Many youngsters in Mattis's classroom have bellies that strain the fabric of their T-shirts or spill over the waistbands of tight jeans. Mattis, an active woman in her early thirties, sometimes takes her students on hikes or field trips. She says she is shocked by their poor stamina. On this Monday morning Mattis has asked her class to write down everything they ate on Saturday. Except for orange juice at breakfast, only 2 of the 27 students list a single fruit. Vegetables, other than French fries, are also rarely mentioned; a few youngsters list salad, broccoli, or squash.

One boy writes, "Breakfast: pizza, chips, cereal, ice cream, donuts. Lunch: pizza, cupcakes, Cheetos. Dinner: pizza, soup, bread. Snacks: pizza, chips, sugar."

A girl writes, "Breakfast: none. Lunch: hot dogs. Dinner: rice, beans, hamburger, macaroni salad. Snacks: chips, soda, ice cream, cupcake, gum."

During the lesson, Mattis's students are surprised to learn that being overweight is causing health problems for kids, but when I ask them what they think might be causing an obesity epidemic in American children, they come up with plenty of theories. Their top suggestions: junk food, fast foods, candy, soda. The discussion turns to physical activity. Most of the children tell me they live close enough to walk to school. In their physical education classes, the school's playing field is so crowded with students, and teachers are so few, that many kids spend the period standing or sitting on the sidelines.

I ask them why they suppose that kids might be getting less exercise than they did 20 years ago.

"Technology."

"Too lazy."

"Crime."

"Traffic."

"Some don't like to go outside and play," offers one boy. "They're depressed."

Just as the cause of the deadly respiratory illness SARS was unknown when it emerged in China and triggered an international epidemic in 2003, the cause of the obesity epidemic is a mystery so far. However, many people claim to know why it is happening. They look at their children's lifestyles and point to super-sized sodas, TV and video games, and snack foods. They look at their own habits and blame their weight problem on eating too much fast food, too many sweets, or spending too much time in their cars. Chances are, they are partly right: all of these factors are likely contributors.

Americans of all backgrounds and socioeconomic groups share many aspects of the modern lifestyle: Meagan and Christine Mattis's students like to eat sweets and high-fat snacks, sit for hours each week in front of computers or TV sets, and spend too little time playing outside. Still, no one knows for certain which aspects of our modern environment—which of the many and complex changes in most people's diet and lifestyles during recent decades—have played the greatest role in unleashing the epidemic of excess body fat that now threatens the future health of children and adults in the United States and elsewhere.

Scientists can at least state with confidence that the causes are environmental, because 25 or 30 years is far too short a time for millions of people all over the planet to have acquired some new genetic mutation that is making them fat. Something about modern life is apparently making increasing numbers of children and adults take in more calories as fuel than they burn during their daily activities, so that the excess is being stored on their bodies as unhealthy quantities of fat. The human body has evolved extremely precise mechanisms to maintain a balance between the energy it consumes as food and the energy it expends to function and move around. It has a set of sensors and signals that keep its weight exquisitely stable over the months and years. Yet the rapid rate of change occurring in today's environment, propelled by our actions, seems to have outpaced the human body's ability to adapt. Our internal weight-regulating mechanisms, which evolved during our species' long history of privation in order to protect us from starvation, have rendered us ill suited for a lifestyle that offers an abundant supply of calories and too little opportunity for physical activity.

All the same, researchers have not pinpointed which aspects of the modern environment are most responsible for rising rates of obesity. They haven't even ruled out the possibility that the epidemic might be caused by a virus or a toxin that affects nerve cells in the brain that regulate appetite. Although such an explanation is considered highly unlikely, compared with the myriad and obvious forces in the environment that encourage people to eat more and to move around less, in the words of obesity scientist Rudy Leibel of Columbia University, "It's a formal possibility."

🐾🐾🐾

Even the words we use to talk about obesity make it difficult to confront the realities of the epidemic in children. "Obesity" is an accepted medical term when applied to adults, but pediatricians shy away from the word, perceiving it as pejorative. In pediatric journals and treatment guidelines, doctors who study and treat children use the term "overweight" rather than "obese." I visited a specialty clinic dedicated to treating obese children that was euphemistically named the "fitness clinic." Because fatness is considered unattractive in mainstream American culture, many people, when discussing their own obesity or that of family members, avoid words like "obese," "fat," or "overweight" in favor of words they consider more tactful, such as "big" or "heavy."

The language used by medical professionals and the public reflects unspoken social and cultural attitudes about obesity, particularly the belief that obese individuals are fat through their own fault, because they lack willpower or self-control. As I will explain in the next chapter, this belief is false.

Euphemisms prevent us from facing the situation. Americans must accept that the obesity epidemic, especially in children, is a public health emergency. To learn about it and figure out how we should respond, we need to use language that is clear and easy to understand. In 2005 a group of experts recruited by the nonprofit Institute of Medicine (IOM) of the National Academies, in Washington, D.C., offered recommendations to the federal government, policymakers, and the general public on how to prevent obesity in children. In issuing their report—*Preventing Childhood Obesity: Health in the Balance*—these experts consciously chose to use the word "obese" rather than "overweight." (Throughout this book I use these two words interchangeably when discussing children who have unhealthy levels of body fat.)

What standards are used to decide whether a person is overweight? Healthy weights for children and adults have been determined by studying large population samples. Weight is not necessarily a direct measurement of body fat stores, since our bodies are made up of bone, muscle, and other tissues as well as fat. However, since it is expensive and impractical to measure body fat stores in large numbers of people, researchers and health care workers have chosen a surrogate measurement that correlates reasonably well with fat stores in all but the most muscular people. A figure called the body mass index, or BMI, has been adopted as a practical tool for determining whether a person's weight (adjusted for height) falls within the range of weights considered to be healthy. The BMI is calculated by dividing weight in kilograms by the square of the height in meters. Charts or BMI calculators, available on the Internet, make it easy to look up the BMI that corresponds to a particular height and weight.

In studies of adults, much research data support the concept that certain BMIs fall within the healthy range while others are associated with a higher-than-average risk of illness and death. Adults who have a BMI of 30 or higher are considered "obese" and those with a BMI between 25 and 29 "overweight" because the risk of many diseases, as well as overall mortality, rises with increasing BMI, especially with BMIs above 30.

For children there are not enough data to define precisely what level of fatness begins to pose health risks or whether that level varies depending on a child's age. The situation is complicated by the fact that as long as a child is growing, his or her BMI is a moving target: it changes continually as height and weight change. For this reason, in children, obesity (or, as pediatricians call it, overweight) is defined as a BMI that is higher than the 95th percentile for children of the same age and sex.

To establish a standard range of BMIs for children of different ages, the federal Centers for Disease Control and Prevention developed growth charts using national survey data collected during decades before the childhood obesity epidemic in the United States reached its present level of severity. When BMI measurements of a large group of same-aged boys and girls are plotted on a graph, the resulting distribution curve is roughly bell shaped. The majority of the children represented have BMIs that fall somewhere in the middle of the range, and a minority have BMIs that fall toward the extremes.

Health professionals use the CDC growth charts to determine how a child's BMI compares with those of other children of the same age and sex. A girl's BMI is said to be at the 50th percentile if 50 percent of girls her age have lower BMIs and 50 percent have higher BMIs. If a boy's BMI is at the 90th percentile for his age, it means that 90 percent of boys his age have lower BMIs and only 10 percent have higher ones. For U.S. children, obesity is defined as a BMI that is higher than the 95th percentile. Children whose BMIs fall between the 85th and the 95th percentiles are considered "at risk" of obesity or overweight, which means their weight is high enough to warrant concern and possible medical treatment.

To understand the obesity epidemic in America's children, consider what has been happening to the curve representing BMI distribution during the past few decades. For children of both sexes and every age group, *average* BMI has increased significantly since the 1960s. But that shift in the average BMI value doesn't mean that *all* kids in today's population are heavier than kids were in the 1960s. Rather, most of the change in the curve has occurred on the right-hand side (heavier side) of the bell, which has shifted toward heavier weights, making the downward slope less steep and pushing the curve's end farther to the right. This means that children represented by the "heavy" half of the curve have gotten heavier, while the leaner children represented by the "light" half have remained about the same. This general pattern also holds true for adolescents.

Not only are more American children and adolescents obese than in the past, but the fattest kids in the U.S. population are much more obese than ever before. These changes are not explained by immigra-

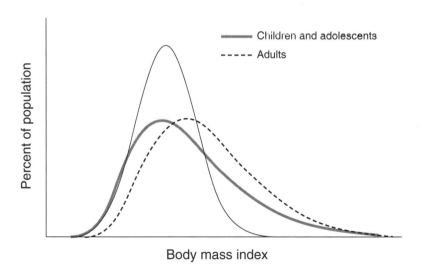

This schematic graph, although not based on actual data, helps illustrate the concept of BMI distribution shifts. The fine solid line represents a standard bell curve, where the curve's peak represents the largest cluster of individuals. As BMI increases or decreases from this mean (midpoint), the number of individuals decreases. As seen by the dashed line, adults have grown heavier, on average, over time; but generally speaking for children and adolescents, heavy youth have grown heavier, while leaner youth have remained more or less at the same weight.

tion or other factors that have produced shifts in the racial or ethnic makeup of the population. Obesity is becoming more prevalent in all racial and ethnic groups, and the increase in prevalence seen among non-Hispanic white children is as large as that seen in other groups.

One way of interpreting the change in the shape of the bell is to say that our modern environment is "obesigenic": it's making an increasingly large fraction of the population gain too much body fat, and it's making that weight gain begin at younger ages. Children whose genes make them moderately vulnerable to obesity, children who probably would not have been overweight in the United States of the 1970s, are becoming overweight today. And those kids with the greatest genetic vulnerability to obesity, who probably would have been fat back then, are gaining much more body fat in today's environment than they would have in the past. This shift toward greater degrees of fatness may help to explain why diseases that were once considered "adult-onset" complications of obesity are now showing up in so many children.

The pattern is somewhat different for adults. The BMI distribution curve for adults has shifted entirely to the right, meaning that virtually the whole population has been affected. Men and women of all ages tend to be heavier today than U.S. adults were during the 1960s. But as in children, the increases in BMI in recent decades have been most dramatic among those adults whose BMI falls on the "heaviest" part of the curve, meaning that the number of severely obese adults in the population has greatly increased.

"We don't really know the magnitude of the health effects here, because we have never before in history had a population that was this overweight," notes obesity researcher Steven L. Gortmaker of the Harvard School of Public Health.

Because being obese threatens the health of affected children, part of our nation's response to the epidemic must include more aggressive efforts by health workers to identify, counsel, and treat children (and the families of those children) who are already overweight or who are at risk of becoming so. Treatment for obesity is more likely to succeed in children than in adolescents or adults, especially if it is started early, before a child has become very overweight. But the childhood obesity epidemic cannot be reversed by relying on medical treatment alone. It's easy to understand why if we consider once again what's been happening to the bell-shaped curve of children's BMIs. The increasing trend toward unhealthy weight gain already affects a sizeable percentage of U.S. children; it is a populationwide phenomenon caused by common factors in our environment, and fixing it will require a populationwide response. Simply focusing on treatment for those kids who are already obese, although vitally important, will not be enough to halt the epidemic, because the percentage of children who are overweight has been rising steadily and that trend shows no sign of slowing down. For every overweight child who is treated, additional children will become obese, eventually overwhelming treatment resources. To halt or reverse the epidemic, we must focus on preventing obesity by favorably changing the environment for all children—for those who are already overweight and for those who are not.

Our desire for a just and equitable society is also a compelling reason for taking populationwide measures. Children of various racial and ethnic groups show dramatically different obesity rates, even though (as I mentioned previously) the prevalence of obesity has been increasing steadily for all groups. This fact probably reflects differences in genetic vulnerability to weight gain, as well as social and cultural differences in children's environments. For example, 46 percent of African American girls aged 12 to 19 are overweight or at risk of becoming so, compared with 25 percent of white girls in the same age group. Among kids of both sexes between the ages of 6 and 11, 40 percent of Mexican Americans and 36 percent of African Americans are overweight or at risk of becoming overweight, compared with 30 percent of whites. The prevalence of obesity among 7-year-old American Indian children is estimated to be almost 30 percent, about twice as high as the prevalence among all U.S. 7-year-olds. These large differences are linked to similarly large ethnic and racial disparities in the risk in adulthood of developing diabetes, high blood pressure, cardiovascular disease, and other obesity-related illnesses. In our obesity prevention efforts we must pay special attention to children who belong to racial and ethnic groups at highest risk.

A child's chances of becoming overweight also appear to be greater if that child is poor. Obesity rates among adults in the United States have increased most rapidly during recent decades in states with the lowest per capita income. Among women, food insecurity (being unsure of having enough to eat, or not having enough of the kinds of food desired) has been shown to be linked with being overweight. Foods that are "energy-dense," providing many calories per pound because of their high sugar or high fat content, are much cheaper than non-energy-dense foods such as fresh fruits, fresh vegetables, and whole grains—the very foods recommended as the basis of an optimally healthy diet. Processed foods also have a longer shelf life than fresh ones. Epidemiologist Adam Drewnowski of the University of Washington argues convincingly that the higher rates of obesity seen among poor populations may reflect the fact that it is far cheaper to eat an unhealthy diet of predominantly energy-dense foods, high in fats and sugars, than it is to eat a "healthy" diet. However, it's probably much more difficult to avoid ingesting too many calories on the energy-dense diet. In addition, low-income neighborhoods often lack access to supermarkets, farmers markets, and other sources of fresh, unprocessed foods, and children in such neighborhoods may not have safe places to go to burn off extra calories through physical activity.

What does the future hold for our nation's children if we do not act to halt the obesity epidemic? Obesity in adults is the number two preventable cause of death in the United States, second only to tobacco use. During the 1990s researchers estimated the annual number of deaths attributable to obesity and lack of physical activity at about 300,000. In the face of steadily rising obesity rates, epidemiologists at the CDC published an updated estimate in 2004 that placed the annual toll of obesity and inactivity at 400,000 deaths per year—and predicted that obesity would soon overtake smoking as the nation's leading cause of preventable death. Although other researchers have criticized the statistical methods used to arrive at this revised estimate, obesity is clearly a major contributor to preventable illness and death.

The direct and indirect medical costs of obesity currently consume about 10 percent of the U.S. health care budget, a percentage that is expected to continue to rise. Overweight people have high rates of diabetes, high cholesterol, high blood pressure, atherosclerotic heart disease, gallbladder disease, and osteoarthritis. Almost 80 percent of obese adults in the United States have one of those conditions, and almost 40 percent have two or more. Obesity is also a risk factor for stroke, congestive heart failure, liver disease, musculoskeletal problems, several kinds of cancer, breathing disorders such as asthma and sleep apnea, and infertility in women, as well as for depression and other psychiatric illnesses.

Until recently, most of our knowledge of the medical consequences of being overweight has come from studies of adults. But in the past two decades, doctors treating the growing numbers of fat children in our society have begun to find cases of what were formerly considered "adult" obesity-related diseases occurring in overweight teenagers and even in kids as young as 6 or 7 years old. The cost of hospitalizations of children aged 6 to 17 for obesity-related illnesses tripled between 1979 and 1999. Meanwhile, a growing body of epidemiological research suggests that childhood obesity by itself may shorten a person's life expectancy, whether or not the individual remains obese as an adult. Such findings underscore the urgency of intervening to prevent obesity in children and treating it when it is present, in order to maximize children's chances of living a long and healthy life.

More than any other factor, it is the rapid rise in type 2 diabetes among children and teenagers that has awakened doctors and health officials to the grim future consequences of the obesity epidemic. In just 12 years, between 1982 and 1994, the incidence of this type of diabetes in children rose tenfold, according to a report by Cincinnati researchers. Type 2 diabetes is a consequence of obesity. Once rare in children, this kind of diabetes now accounts for at least one-third of new cases of diabetes in adolescents—and in some populations up to one-half of new cases. Thirty percent of boys and 40 percent of girls born in the United States in 2000 will become diabetic at some point in their lives unless current obesity trends are reversed, according to projections by epidemiologists at the CDC. Among African American and Hispanic children, almost half will develop diabetes.

Diabetes is a disease in which the body doesn't produce enough insulin, a critically important hormone that regulates the concentration of blood sugar (glucose)—the body's major source of energy—

and directs its use and storage by tissues such as liver and muscle. Unlike someone with type 1 or "childhood" diabetes, a person with type 2 diabetes still makes some insulin, but having too much stored fat renders the body insensitive to the hormone's effects. Type 2 diabetes develops in part because this extra fat tissue puts excessive demands on the body to make insulin, resulting in "insulin resistance." When insulin resistance occurs, specialized cells in the pancreas called beta cells must churn out extra-high levels of the hormone in response to the rise in blood glucose that takes place when a person eats. Eventually the beta cells can't make enough insulin to lower the blood glucose level to within the normal range. Chronically high glucose levels ultimately destroy beta cells, the only cells that can manufacture insulin. Over a period of years, type 2 diabetes causes just as much mayhem to tissues as type 1 diabetes. In both types, high blood glucose levels and other metabolic abnormalities eventually produce damage to blood vessels and nerves, sometimes leading to blindness, kidney failure, heart attack, stroke, and amputation of the feet or legs. Indeed, type 2 diabetes may be a more rapidly progressive disease in children than in adults. Because the frequency of complications is also related to the duration of the disease, experts fear that many obese youngsters now developing type 2 diabetes may suffer heart attacks or other complications by the time they reach their forties.

Although the increase in type 2 diabetes drew attention to the potential impact of the obesity epidemic on children's health, diabetes is only one component in a web of linked derangements of metabolism that obesity can produce in a child or an adult. Doctors and researchers use the term "metabolic syndrome" to refer to a pattern of abnormalities that often occur together. The metabolic syndrome includes five possible features: abdominal obesity, high blood pressure, glucose intolerance (a prediabetic condition in which insulin levels, although high, are insufficient to handle glucose normally), a high blood level of triglycerides (a fat present in the circulation), and a low blood level of high-density lipoprotein or HDL cholesterol (sometimes nicknamed "good" cholesterol because it helps protect against blood vessel damage). A person who has at least three of these five features is said to have the metabolic syndrome.

Having too much fat tissue contributes to development of the metabolic syndrome. Fat cells, once considered inert little bags of oil, have been discovered to make an array of hormones used to communicate with the brain and with other tissues and organs. Some stored fat is necessary for health, but an excess of it, particularly in certain locations, can be life-threatening. Visceral fat, located inside the abdominal cavity, is considered the most metabolically active fat in the body. It produces a somewhat different mix of hormones than fat tissue found elsewhere, and the chemical messages it releases into the circulation travel directly to the liver and other nearby organs, influencing their function.

Research evidence now suggests that disorders such as diabetes, high blood pressure, and heart disease, instead of being separate and unrelated problems, are really interconnected diseases that can all be caused by the metabolic syndrome. Even several years before developing overt diabetes, many obese children already have undiagnosed glucose intolerance as well as other features of the syndrome. Almost 30 percent of overweight children between the ages of 12 and 19 in the United States, and about 4 percent of all U.S. teenagers, have the metabolic syndrome, according to a recent study of a national sample of adolescents. The syndrome is also appearing in younger kids: in fact, doctors who treat pediatric obesity have diagnosed the metabolic syndrome in children as young as 5 years old.

In parallel with the nationwide increases in obesity and in metabolic syndrome, a recent national study found that between 1988 and 2000 the average blood pressure of children in the United States edged upward by a couple of points, a seemingly small shift that nevertheless places many more kids at risk of developing high blood pressure as young adults. Researchers have also documented worrisome changes in the hearts and arteries of obese children, including thickening of the walls of carotid arteries—large vessels that supply blood to the brain—in children as young as 9 years old. Findings such as these may be early warnings of a future surge in adult cases of heart attack, stroke, kidney failure, and other illnesses that seem an almost inevitable consequence of the current epidemic of obesity in children. Some experts have speculated that today's kids may be the first American generation to live shorter lives, on average, than their parents.

Once a boy or girl is overweight, what are the chances of ultimately becoming a lean adult? And what's the evidence that being fat as a child does any lasting damage to health?

Not all fat children grow up to be fat adults. In addition, overweight kids are not all at equal risk of developing medical problems. An overweight child's risk of adult obesity, as well as his or her risk of diabetes, high blood pressure, or other disorders, varies depending on the child's age, racial or ethnic background, and other factors, particularly whether one or both parents are obese and whether there is a family history of obesity-related illnesses.

In the United States today, most obese adults were not obese as children. About two-thirds of people who are overweight or obese as adults were not overweight during the first 20 years of their lives. That pattern may change in the future, however, since so many more children are overweight today. A key 1997 study examined the risk of adult obesity for kids who were fat at different ages. It found that among children under 3 years old, being fat by itself does not significantly increase the likelihood of becoming a fat adult. But after the age of 3, the older an obese child is, the greater the likelihood that obesity will persist. After age 6, the probability of an obese child becoming an obese adult is greater than 50 percent, compared with about 10 percent for non-obese children. The risk of adult obesity rises higher for kids who are obese after the age of 10. In addition, the more overweight a child is, the greater the chance of being obese as an adult.

Having one obese parent also was found to multiply a child's risk of adult obesity about twofold to threefold, compared to that of a child with two lean parents. If both parents are obese, the child's risk is further increased. The authors of the study suggest that children between the ages of 3 and 9 who are overweight, especially those who have at least one obese parent, "may be ideal candidates for treatment because the parents still have the opportunity to influence their children's activity and diet positively." A child of any age and body weight whose parents are both obese should probably receive particular attention in order to establish a healthy diet and physical activity habits before obesity develops.

How does being fat affect a child's life expectancy? Clearly, part of the answer depends on whether obesity persists into adulthood, since the longer a person is significantly overweight as an adult, the greater the risk of medical complications such as heart disease, diabetes, and cancer. But a growing body of research indicates that childhood obesity by itself may shorten life span.

The Harvard Growth Study described death rates and disease patterns during the course of a half-century in 508 people who had enrolled in the study as teenagers between 1922 and 1935. At enrollment they were classified as "lean" if their BMI fell between the 25th and 50th percentiles; if it was greater than the 75th percentile, they were classified as "overweight." Among the men in this study—but not the women—being overweight as a teenager was associated with a higher mortality rate in adulthood from all causes. The men who had been overweight as adolescents had a death rate almost twice as high as those who had been lean, and their death rate from heart disease was more than double that of their lean counterparts. The frequency of heart disease was greater in both sexes among people who had been overweight as teenagers. The men who had been overweight adolescents had higher rates of colon cancer and gout; the women had higher rates of arthritis. These findings were independent of adult weight. In other words, people's risk of developing these diseases was more closely linked to whether they had been fat as teenagers than to whether they were fat as adults. The sex difference in mortality rates seen in the Harvard Growth Study is puzzling but may only be a statistical artifact.

Recently a much larger study found that being overweight in adolescence affects adult mortality rates about equally in both sexes. In that study, Norwegian researchers tracked the health of 227,003 adolescents aged 14 to 19, whose height and weight were measured between 1963 and 1975. Participants were followed for an average of 31 years. Men and women whose BMI as teenagers fell between the 85th and 95th percentiles (a category U.S. pediatricians currently term "at risk of overweight") had a death rate as adults that was 30 percent higher than that seen in people of the same sex who had been lean adolescents (BMI between the 25th and 75th percentiles). Among women whose BMI as teenagers was above the 95th percentile (classified under current U.S. pediatric standards as "overweight") the adult death rate was twice that of women who had been lean; among men who had been similarly overweight as teenagers, the adult death rate was almost twice as high as for men who had been lean. Interestingly, the difference in death rates remained small and not statistically significant while participants were in their twenties. The impact of adolescent overweight on adult death rates did not become sizeable until study participants were between 30 and 58 years old.

This study offers powerful evidence that being fat in the teenage years has a lifelong effect on health. The finding of higher death rates among people who had been overweight teenagers was independent of participants' adult weight. Since deaths among young adults are rare, it required a very large and carefully conducted study, lasting for decades, to show this impact. The Norwegian study had remarkably complete follow-up: out of more than 227,000 participants, the status of only 33 was unknown at the study's end. However, the researchers were unable to collect information about causes of death or about other potential risk factors such as smoking, lack of exercise, and socioeconomic class.

So far it has been difficult for researchers to determine whether the impact of obesity on life expectancy differs among racial and ethnic groups. One recent study of U.S. mortality data concluded that being severely obese as a young adult reduces life expectancy more in black men than in white men, but more in white women than in black women. These findings, however, have been criticized on various technical grounds (for instance, failure to make statistical adjustments for lower socioeconomic status, which also reduces life expectancy). As yet, few studies have addressed the same question for Hispanic Americans or American Indians, although these groups have a high incidence of obesity and diabetes.

What is clear, though, is that obesity increases the risk of many specific diseases, such as diabetes and high blood pressure, in people of all racial and ethnic groups. Conversely, weight loss has been shown to reduce the risk of diabetes, high blood pressure, and various other diseases among overweight people of all racial and ethnic backgrounds who are not yet sick and to improve health for those who already have such disorders.

Bruce and his mother, Lottie, have radically changed their family's environment. They did it a few months ago, after Bruce, who is African American, was diagnosed at age 18 with high blood pressure and was sent by his pediatrician to a Charlottesville, Virginia, clinic that helps children lose weight. Obesity runs in Bruce's father's family, and Lottie considered Bruce's diagnosis a wake-up call. Bruce and his mother and sisters still live in the same small brick house in a modest neighborhood on the east side of town. And Bruce, a shy, round-faced boy with oval glasses, still goes to technical school each day, studying to get his high school degree and be certified as an auto mechanic. But the dishes in the cupboards, the snacks and drinks in the refrigerator, and the family routines—even the way the kids watch television—are all new.

Lottie gave away her tall glasses and bought short ones that hold only 8 ounces. She bought plastic plates that are subdivided into three sections, with the biggest section—occupying half of the surface area—reserved for vegetables. She stopped purchasing fried potato chips and corn chips, opting instead for rice cakes and single-serving cups of nonfat yogurt with fruit. She switched to low-fat milk and diet sodas instead of regular soft drinks, and she stocks up on fresh fruit, whole wheat bread, and multigrain cereal. She's cut back on trips to fast food restaurants and orders pizza only on rare occasions.

At the clinic, the dietician gave Bruce a pedometer to clip onto his belt so he could count the number of steps he took each day. He started walking up and down the stairs during commercials while watching television to try to reach his daily goal of 7,000 steps. He began working out on the family's manual treadmill or doing aerobics along with the exercise shows. His older sister, Latoya, enticed him outside on sunny afternoons to shoot baskets at the hoop up the street. Sometimes Lottie and all three of her children went to the local high school and walked around the track.

During the first month in his new home environment, Bruce lost 6 pounds. His mother and sisters lost weight too. In the months since, Bruce has continued to lose fat and to add muscle. His blood pressure has come down. Even more important, the foods and drinks he chooses, his portion sizes, and his exercise habits have all been transformed—probably for good. He no longer eats French fries or drinks soda for lunch at school. He still hates to run around in hot weather, but he has far more energy and he has slimmed down so much his mother had to buy him a new wardrobe.

What is heartening about Bruce's story, and about the stories of other families whose children are being treated at the Charlottesville clinic, is that they prove it's not really so hard to change an overweight child's environment and to see big improvements in habits and overall health. Bruce's experience is not unique. Staff members at the clinic say that as they monitor their young patients, they see pants sizes changing and laboratory results improving even before kids' weights start to go down. Simply providing a better diet and getting children to be more physically active is enough to start to build stronger bodies and reverse some of the incipient medical problems caused by excess weight.

Most parents are eager to take action when told their child is sick. It's much more difficult to persuade families to make major alterations in their lifestyle when children seem to be well, merely to prevent disease sometime in the future. Yet that's what we must do. When doctors and public health officials tell us that almost one-third of our children are sick with obesity or are at risk of becoming so, it's time for us to change our children's environment, both inside and outside the home, in ways that will help them build leaner and healthier bodies.

Changing the environment for our entire society will mean changing prevailing attitudes and social norms in much the way they have changed with regard to smoking. Addressing the obesity epidemic will be much more complicated than that of tobacco-related illness, however. For tobacco, the solution was obvious: simply reduce the percentage of people who smoke, chew, or sniff the substance. Still, there is a positive side to the fact that there appear to be many contributors to the increase in childhood obesity. It means there are many ways of taking action to improve children's habits and environment. Even as we wait for clearer scientific answers to the question of which factors are most responsible, we can act on the information we already have to try to improve the health outlook for all children.

Preventing Childhood Obesity: Health in the Balance, the 2005 IOM report, contains a road map for action at home, at school, in the community, and at both state and national levels. For parents, key recommendations include providing healthy food choices and modeling healthy eating; encouraging children to be physically active for at least an hour a day and maximizing the time they spend outside; and carefully limiting how much time kids spend watching television or using computers and video games. It advises that *all* foods and beverages sold or served in schools meet new government nutritional standards and recommends the overall improvement of their nutritional quality. In addition, schools should provide a minimum of 30 minutes of moderate to vigorous physical activity and expand opportunities for kids to play sports and be active both at school and in child-care or after-school programs. The report endorses efforts to make neighborhoods more walkable, bikeable, and exercise-friendly and to promote broader access to fresh, healthy foods and to exercise or recreation facilities, especially for children and adolescents in urban or low-income communities that often lack such resources.

It also calls for campaigns on the local and national levels to educate children and teenagers about how to make healthy dietary choices and about the importance of daily activity. And it sounds alarms about the potential long-term damage being done to children's health by our nation's food industry through ubiquitous, child-targeted marketing and advertising of high-calorie, high-sugar, and high-fat foods and drinks, and by the entertainment industry's promotion of video games, television shows, and other sedentary activities. It recommends the development and implementation of new national guidelines to reduce the role of such advertising in promoting childhood obesity and calls on Congress to give the Federal Trade Commission (FTC) the authority and funds to monitor advertisers' compliance with such guidelines.

In this book I provide an overview of current scientific understanding about what factors in the environment are contributing to the epidemic of obesity in children and offer suggestions about what parents and other adults can do to prevent kids from becoming overweight. In the next chapter I explain what we know about genetic vulnerability to obesity and about how the human body regulates its appetite and energy expenditure to maintain a constant weight.

Chapter 3 examines the complicated relationship between children's weight (or BMI) and body image, as well as the effect of being overweight on a child's mood and relationships with other kids. It includes advice for parents and others on how to address a child's weight as a medical issue without damaging self-esteem.

Chapters 4 and 5 focus on fostering healthy eating habits in kids and on promoting physical activity. Chapter 6 explores recent evidence that children's food preferences, calorie intake, and even their bodies' innate ability to regulate weight and appetite are influenced by their environment in the uterus before birth, as well as by choices that parents make regarding breastfeeding and infant feeding during the first year of life.

Chapter 7 deals with making our schools a healthier environment for children and especially describes efforts to make the kinds of food and drink sold at schools more consistent with the nutrition lessons that are being taught in classrooms.

Chapter 8 offers information on finding good treatment for an overweight child, including specialized programs for children who are severely obese. It also examines the ongoing debate about the long-term risks and benefits of weight-loss surgery and about whether such procedures should be made available, in certain cases, to adolescents.

Chapter 9, the last chapter, suggests ways people can work to prevent obesity at the community, state, or national level. It is followed by a list of resources for readers who want to explore opportunities for political action or learn more about specific aspects of childhood obesity.

If we do not try to turn back the childhood obesity epidemic the consequences will be dire. As David L. Katz of the Yale School of Medicine puts it, "Children growing up in the United States today will suffer more chronic disease and premature death because of the way they eat and their lack of physical activity than from exposure to tobacco, drugs, and alcohol combined."

If you want to protect children—your own and those of others—from the greatest threat to their future health, start now.

CHAPTER 2

Obese Twins and Thrifty Genes

Rudy Leibel's genes may have predisposed him to become a brilliant scientist, but his decision to spend his life trying to discover the cause of obesity was not predestined. That choice was influenced by an angry mother. Not Leibel's mother, but the mother of a fat boy named Randall. They met in 1977. Rudolph L. Leibel was a rising star on the Harvard Medical School faculty, an assistant professor of pediatrics at Cambridge City Hospital, in Massachusetts. A busy public hospital in a working-class neighborhood, Cambridge City received its share of tough pediatric cases: children with meningitis, toddlers with bones broken by abusive parents, teenagers who had attempted suicide. Leibel, a scholarly young doctor who favored neat bow ties and fashionably long hair, was revered by the hospital's pediatric residents for his ingenious rescues of seemingly hopeless cases.

The residents liked to recount the story of one young patient who had tried to kill himself by taking an overdose of chloroquine, a drug prescribed to travelers to prevent malaria. Leibel consulted a toxicology textbook and found the prognosis grim: doses in the range that the boy had swallowed were uniformly fatal because the drug impaired the functioning of the heart's natural pacemaker. Within hours of such an overdose, the victim invariably died from cardiac arrest. Leibel persuaded the director of the adult cardiac care unit to admit the child, who at that point still seemed fine, and to hook him up to an electronic heart monitor. He arranged to have a cardiologist stand by, and then he waited at the bedside. When the boy's heart suddenly stopped several hours later, Leibel and a medical team promptly administered CPR, threaded a pacemaker into the patient's heart, and started it up again. The case became a hospital legend.

But in the spring of 1977 Rudy Leibel encountered a child he couldn't rescue. Randall was a severely overweight boy whose mother had brought him to be examined by the young professor, who specialized in hormone disorders. Leibel could find no evidence of a hormone deficiency or of any other known medical cause of Randall's obesity; the boy was simply fat. When he told Randall's mother there was little he or anyone could do for her son, she erupted.

"Let's get out of here, Randall," she snapped, heading for the door. "This doctor doesn't know shit."

A quarter of a century later, doctors know quite a bit more about obesity—thanks in part to the gauntlet thrown down by Randall's mother. Chastened by her words, Leibel soon traded his post as a Harvard professor for the low-paying toil of a rookie laboratory scientist, moving his family to New York and taking a job in the Rockefeller University laboratory of Jules Hirsch, an eminent obesity researcher. He and Hirsch performed extensive studies, expanding on work by other scientists, that detailed how the body responds either to weight gain or to weight loss by fighting to restore the status quo. In one of these studies, volunteers were induced to overeat until they gained weight. This proved a remarkably difficult task for Leibel's research subjects, fat or lean, because their bodies responded by turning up their metabolic rates, boosting the levels of certain hormones, reducing hunger, and burning up more calories as heat—all in an unconscious but coordinated effort to get back to the original weight. If people's intake was restricted so that they lost weight, their bodies fought back even more fiercely. Their metabolism slowed, they moved around less, their muscles burned fewer calories when they exercised, and they felt constantly and uncomfortably hungry. A host of physiological defense mechanisms swung into play, aimed at regaining the lost pounds.

Findings like these persuaded Leibel that such tight physiological regulation of body weight must mean that the brain was receiving a chemical signal from the body's fat stores. That conviction ultimately led to the discovery of leptin, a hormone produced by fat cells that became the key to a new biological understanding of how appetite and weight are controlled. Animal studies proved that leptin was the long-sought molecular message that traveled through the circulatory system from fat cells to the brain, signaling that energy stores were sufficient and that it was safe to stop eating. Mice that were genetically incapable of producing leptin ate nonstop and grew enormously tubby. Treating such mice with leptin normalized their body weight.

When the gene for leptin was identified and sequenced in 1994 as a result of an intensive collaborative effort between Leibel and Jeffrey M. Friedman of Rockefeller University, many people (and some drug companies) predicted that the newly identified hormone would become a miracle cure for obesity. They assumed that fat people must be lacking in leptin and that dosing them with it would make them lose weight. It has not turned out that way. Most obese people make plenty of their own leptin, but for unknown reasons their brains are relatively resistant to the hormone's effects, so that even large doses don't work very well as a weight-loss drug. Recent findings by Leibel and others suggest, however, that leptin may have a future role as a treatment that helps people keep weight off after they've lost large amounts. A fall in leptin levels occurs with loss of body fat and seems to trigger the physiological changes that make people regain lost pounds, so boosting leptin levels after weight loss may help prevent that gain.

The discovery of leptin transformed the science of obesity by persuading the research community that obesity had a biological basis. Almost overnight, hundreds of talented scientists the world over became eager to investigate how appetite and weight are regulated. Scores of papers on the subject are now published each year, and every few months another small but important piece of the immensely complicated genetic and biological puzzle falls into place; another hormone or cellular receptor is pinpointed as a possible target for future new treatments.

Leibel—his hair now gray and cropped short, his bowtie and button-down shirt replaced by a soft crewneck sweater—heads a laboratory that occupies two floors of a gleaming new research building in upper Manhattan, filled with gene-sequencing equipment and cages of mice and staffed by industrious young scientists. As director of molecular genetics at Columbia University, he and his group are working to identify the major genes that make so many people dangerously prone to obesity and to one of its frequent consequences, diabetes.

What would he say to Randall's mother now? To begin with, if she walked into his office today, he'd be able to assure her that Randall's problem was in large measure biological, and not simply the result of faulty parenting or lack of willpower. "There really is a biology to the regulation of body weight, just as there is a biology to the regulation of height or blood pressure or eye color," Leibel says. "I would say to her, 'Randall has a disorder of a regulatory system that is important for the control of weight.'"

The years since the discovery of leptin have been hailed as a golden age for obesity research. In little more than a decade, scientists have sketched the broad outlines of the biological system that regulates body weight and have begun filling in the details. The control centers for tracking energy balance and regulating body weight are located primarily in the hypothalamus, a small part of the brain that specializes in integrating messages from many parts of the body and orchestrating the organism's response to its environment. The hypothalamus communicates by nerve pathways and chemical signals with many other brain areas, as well as with the organs that make up the cardiovascular system, the digestive system, the reproductive system, and the endocrine system (the glands that produce circulating hormones). It uses its output both to modify conscious, purposeful behavior such as food-seeking and to fine-tune unconscious processes such as metabolism, reproductive cycles and the level of arousal, and spontaneous physical activity. Leibel points out that unconscious signals sent by the hypothalamus to the cerebral cortex, the "thinking" part of the brain, thus contribute to such conscious actions as ordering a pizza or having a second piece of pie. "Just because a behavior is involved does not mean that all aspects of the behavior are 'voluntary' in the usual sense of the word," he says.

Because taking in food and maintaining sufficient energy stores are necessary for survival and reproduction, our bodies are designed to preserve these functions at all costs. The system for maintaining body weight is like a castle surrounded by multiple walls, a computer operating system with many built-in backups, or the redundant controls of a commercial airliner. It evolved to fight starvation, so it is engineered according to the principle that storing too much energy is preferable to storing too little. During most of the several million years of human evolution, a tendency to store extra body fat during times of plenty has bestowed a marked survival advantage. As Leibel observes, if we still lived in the environment of 100,000 years ago, "Randall would be king."

What are the brain's strategies for keeping body weight constant? In issuing its instructions, the hypothalamus can respond to information from the environment in three general ways. It can influence food intake by increasing or decreasing appetite. It can fine-tune the body's metabolic rate—the rate at which it burns calories merely to stay alive—by sending messages to the autonomic nervous system and to endocrine glands such as the thyroid, the insulin-producing cells in the pancreas, and the adrenals, which regulate metabolism. And it can further affect the body's total expenditure of calories by adjusting how much energy is released as heat during certain cellular processes or through muscle activity such as exercise or fidgeting.

The main appetite control center of the hypothalamus is located in an area called the arcuate nucleus. Within it are populations of two different types of nerve cells. One type of cell makes a pair of chemicals—neuropeptide Y or NPY, and agouti-related protein, or AGRP—that transmit signals to other nerve cells to increase appetite. The other type makes a pair of substances—POMC and CART—that relay signals with the opposite effect, decreasing appetite. (The unwieldy names of some of the chemical messengers in this system make it seem more mystifying than it is. POMC stands for proopiomelanocortin; CART stands for cocaine-and-amphetamine-regulated transcript.) These two types of nerve cells communicate with each other, and both types also send opposing messages to a third group of nerve cells that contain a signal-receiving protein on their surfaces called the melanocortin 4 receptor (MC4R). Depending on whether the activity of the NPY/AGRP cells or the POMC/CART cells predominates at a certain time, the net effect is to turn appetite up or down.

The NPY/AGRP cells and POMC/CART cells in the arcuate nucleus do not send their signals at random; they respond to messages coming in via the circulation or nervous system from other parts of the body. These messages convey both long-term information about the status of body energy stores and short-term information, such as the current circulating level of glucose and the presence or absence of food in the intestinal tract. The role of nerve cells in the arcuate nucleus and in related areas of the hypothalamus is to integrate minute-to-minute information on the body's nutritional status and to respond by adjusting food intake and energy use in order to keep body weight constant—in other words, to keep the body in "energy balance."

Where do the messages being sent to the brain originate? Leptin and to a lesser extent insulin carry information about long-term energy depots. Leptin is an emissary from fat tissue, and its level in the circulation reflects how much fat is stored in the body. Leptin's chief function seems to be to protect energy stores and prevent starvation. It also serves as a link between nutritional status and the reproductive system, probably helping to prevent pregnancy if energy stores are inadequate. (Puberty does not occur normally in girls whose bodies do not make leptin, and from puberty onward, women's leptin levels are two to three times higher than men's.)

When an animal's or a person's food intake is severely restricted, leptin levels drop within 24 hours—well before fat stores have been significantly depleted by being burned for energy. The fall in leptin triggers an immediate lowering of the metabolic rate, increased hunger, and a rise in food intake, as well as some suppression of the reproductive and immune systems. These responses seem designed to ward off the threat of starvation by protecting energy stores and cutting back on noncritical energy expenditure. As I mentioned earlier, the body's response to high leptin levels, such as those found in overweight children or adults, is far less dramatic.

Insulin, the hormone produced by the beta cells of the pancreas, is released into the bloodstream in response to glucose from food. It helps direct the body's use and storage of this key fuel, as well as the balance between the storage and burning of fat. Insulin levels fall during fasting and rise in obesity. Some nerve cells in the brain sense and respond to insulin as another signal of overall nutritional status. Some brain cells also respond directly to circulating levels of fuels such as glucose and free fatty acids.

The brain also receives messages from the digestive tract. Constant updates about food availability and the timing of meals are relayed to the hypothalamus by various messenger molecules released by cells in the stomach and intestinal tract. Ghrelin is a recently discovered stomach hormone that signals to the hypothalamus when it is time to eat; it may also help determine the level of hunger. PYY, another signaling molecule, is produced in certain portions of the intestines in response to the arrival of food and apparently informs the brain when it is time to stop eating. A number of other digestive tract hormones are also released in response to nutrients. Some of these signals from the gut may turn out to play important roles in appetite, feeding, and energy balance.

The idea of two opposing groups of nerve cells issuing signals to turn appetite up or down is a simple and elegant concept, but it is nevertheless an incomplete picture of how the brain regulates body weight. Scientists have identified a number of additional chemical transmitters and nerve pathways within the brain that also influence appetite and energy expenditure. For example, nerve cells in an area of the lateral hypothalamus make a substance called melanin concentrating hormone, or MCH, that seems to play a role in the drive to feed. Mice with too much MCH are obese, and mice unable to make MCH are lean, eat little, and burn lots of calories. The nerve cells that produce MCH receive messages from both the appetite-inducing (NPY/ AGRP) cells and the appetite-suppressing (POMC/CART) cells of the arcuate nucleus. Various other signaling chemicals widely present in the brain (and, in some cases, elsewhere in the body) also affect hunger, satiety, metabolic rate, and fat storage, including a family of appetite-boosting brain chemicals called endocannabinoids, related to the active ingredients in marijuana.

Our bodies' elaborate mechanisms for regulating appetite and food intake evolved to ensure survival, but we also eat because food is enjoyable. The pleasure associated with eating may serve as an additional survival mechanism, yet it can also drive humans (and animals) to eat more calories than they need, especially when the food before them looks, smells, and tastes delicious. Human eating behavior is highly influenced too by external cues and routines, by social situations, and by other factors such as mood and stress. Sensory input from smell and taste receptors in the nose and mouth sends signals to many areas of the brain, a fact that helps explain why a specific smell or taste can evoke a flood of feelings, memories, and associations. Imaging studies have shown that when people are presented with appetizing, good-smelling food, many regions of the brain become metabolically active and "light up" on scans.

Scientists know less about the brain pathways and signals that produce the rewarding or comforting sensations of eating than they do about the ones that regulate appetite. A brain area called the nucleus accumbens, implicated as a "reward center" active in drug addiction, is thought to be involved in the pleasure associated with food, although additional brain regions probably also participate. The nucleus accumbens receives input from the cerebral cortex (the "conscious" brain) about sensory and social factors in the environment that influence eating as well as from the areas of the hypothalamus that regulate appetite and feeding. Opioid receptors—the cell-surface proteins that respond to narcotics such as heroin—are thought to be involved in producing the pleasant sensations associated with food. The ubiquitous transmitter chemicals dopamine and serotonin, which relay messages along nerve pathways in many regions of the brain, are also believed to affect feeding behavior and the rewarding aspects of food. The fact that nerve pathways and brain cells associated with pleasure are activated by both food and drugs does not mean that food intake should be considered an "addictive" behavior. As Leibel points out, substances that commonly produce addiction, such as heroin, tobacco, and alcohol, are not critical to survival, but all animals must eat to live.

Hormones arriving from elsewhere in the body can influence the brain's perceptions of food and can even contribute to conscious cravings for certain kinds of foods. For instance, high levels of leptin blunt the perception of sweet tastes. A recent study found that in rats steroid hormones such as corticosterone, released by the adrenal glands in response to chronic stress, stimulated the animals to eat sweet or high-fat food, which calmed them. (Humans whose adrenal glands make too high a level of steroid hormones, or those who take steroids as drugs, also tend to have an increased appetite and may eat more food than they need.) Findings like these may help explain why people who are depressed or anxious often seek out specific "comfort foods."

The result of this complicated dance of signals between the brain and the rest of the body is that human beings, whether lean or obese, eat tens of millions of calories over the course of their lifetimes, burn up most of that energy to stay alive and move around, and tend to keep their body weight remarkably constant at a personal "set point." They store any calories that they do not use up, mostly in the form of fat tissue. However, fat tissue is not just a passive storage depot, like a jar of olive oil sitting in the cupboard. In addition to fat cells, fat tissue contains nerve cells, immune system cells, and other components. As mentioned earlier, fat cells themselves are active performers in the dance of signals, processing fuels and sending out messages, in the form of hormones and other substances, that influence the workings of the brain and other organs and tissues.

Although leptin is the best-known hormone produced by fat cells, there are at least eight or nine others, and the list keeps growing. They include resistin, which interferes with the body's handling of glucose; adiponectin, which promotes glucose utilization and fatty acid oxidation; and various other proteins that influence the immune system, kidney function, and blood clotting. In addition, fat cells actively metabolize steroid hormones such as male and female sex hormones from the reproductive system and glucocorticoids (cortisol and related chemicals) from the adrenal glands. Metabolism and release of steroid hormones by fat cells stored inside the abdominal cavity (visceral fat) is thought by scientists to play a central role in producing the metabolic syndrome—the pattern of abnormalities, described in Chapter 1, that is increasingly occurring in overweight children and that can lead to diabetes, heart disease, and other chronic illnesses.

☙☙☙

If Randall were to become Leibel's patient today, he might undergo testing for a genetic cause of his obesity. A few unlucky people are born with a single genetic mutation that stacks the deck so overwhelmingly that they become severely overweight almost no matter what their environment is. At least five different "obesity genes" have been identified that are so critical to the regulation of appetite and food intake that certain mutations in any one of them can produce extreme obesity. These rare mutations cause "monogenic" or single-gene obesity.

In 1997, three years after the report of the discovery and sequencing of the gene for leptin in mice, a team of British researchers led by Stephen O'Rahilly reported the cases of two children, cousins in a large Pakistani family living in England, who had suffered from severe obesity since infancy. Their brothers and sisters were not overweight. The girl, at the age of 9, weighed 200 pounds and had already undergone an orthopedic operation because her fatness had bowed her leg bones. Her cousin, a boy, weighed 64 pounds as a 2-year-old. Both children had been normal-sized infants at birth but had insatiable appetites. They were not diabetic, and their bodies burned calories at normal rates. Their obesity was chiefly the result of constant eating: their bodies were more than 50 percent fat.

Tests showed that both children had a mutation in the gene for leptin. Their fat cells could not make the hormone, so their brains were not receiving a critical signal needed to regulate their appetites. The pair of cases represented the first discovery of a single-gene cause of obesity in humans. When doctors began giving the cousins regular leptin injections, their food intake fell dramatically and the fat virtually melted off their bodies. Several years later the weights of both children are normal for their ages. The older cousin, now a teenager, progressed normally through puberty like her schoolmates with the help of her leptin treatments.

Without leptin these children—and a few others who have been found to carry the same kind of rare mutation—are unable to transmit messages from their fat cells to their brains about how much energy the body has stored. As a result, they eat voraciously and become obese. So do a few equally rare individuals whose brains cannot sense the presence of leptin because of a mutation in the gene for the leptin receptor, a key docking site for the hormone. A third gene contains the instructions for making an enzyme called prohormone convertase 1 (PC-1), needed for the production of both leptin and insulin, yet another hormone that's an important player in weight regulation. Children with mutations in any of these three genes—the gene for leptin, for the leptin receptor, or for PC-1—are severely obese. Because of leptin's effects on the reproductive system, they also fail to show signs of puberty upon reaching early adolescence, a fact that often leads to the diagnosis of their genetic condition.

A fourth "obesity gene" contains the code for proopiomelanocortin or POMC, a previously mentioned appetite-suppressing chemical made by the hypothalamus. POMC helps regulate not only appetite but the functioning of the adrenal glands (important for salt and fluid balance, metabolism, and stress responses) as well as the body's manufacture of pigments that color the skin and hair. When the gene is mutated, the messenger fails to perform any of its functions, and so children with POMC mutations are overweight and red-haired and have adrenal glands that don't work properly.

Mutations in a fifth gene are by far the most frequent single-gene cause of obesity yet discovered, accounting for up to 5 percent of cases of severe childhood obesity. (Testing so far has been performed mainly in children of European ancestry; such mutations may turn out to be less common in obese children from other ethnic groups.) The affected gene contains instructions for making the cell-surface protein called the melanocortin 4 receptor (MC4R). These receptors, also mentioned earlier, are found on certain nerve cells in the hypothalamus, where they serve as docking sites for signaling chemicals involved in appetite regulation, especially the appetite-suppressing signal derived from POMC. If the cells of the hypothalamus lack functioning MC4R receptors because of a genetic mutation, they cannot sense the signal's presence and appetite is not suppressed. People with this kind of mutation are abnormally hungry: they overeat and become obese. Children with MC4R receptor mutations, besides being heavy, are tall for their age and have unusually dense bones.

In most cases, identifying one of these gene mutations as the cause of an individual's obesity does not mean that a doctor can successfully treat or cure it. Nevertheless, understanding these monogenic causes of very severe obesity has given scientists a precise explanation for what causes the weight problem in people with such mutations and has allowed them to fit together pieces of the puzzle showing how the body regulates food intake and fat stores in individuals without such mutations. Finding additional single-gene causes of obesity is likely to lead eventually to the development of far more effective medical diagnosis and treatments. Mutations in single genes "surely do not represent the majority of instances of human obesity—even severe obesity—from what we can tell now," Leibel says. "But they reinforce this idea that there are single genes that very, very potently and profoundly affect energy balance and body weight in humans."

Most overweight children don't need genetic testing as part of their routine medical care, but those who are severely obese may, especially if obesity has developed at a very young age. Hormone problems and genetic disorders cause far fewer than 10 percent of all cases of childhood obesity. Doctors can measure blood levels of certain hormones—such as leptin or proinsulin—as initial tests that might suggest the presence of some mutations. Obesity is also a feature of certain rare inherited syndromes—constellations of abnormalities caused by single or multiple genes. For example, children with Bardet-Biedl syndrome are very overweight and also frequently have extra fingers or toes, degeneration of the retinas of their eyes, and developmental delays. Children with Prader-Willi syndrome are often scrawny or underweight for the first year or two of their lives, then develop an insatiable appetite and become severely obese; they are also unusually short, have poor muscle tone, and suffer from mental retardation or learning disabilities.

Because Leibel specializes in the genetics of obesity, he regularly receives calls and e-mail messages from doctors around the country who are faced with a seriously overweight youngster and want to know whether they are dealing with one of the known mutations or with some other inherited cause of the condition. If a case seems to fit the profile of one of the genetic forms of obesity, he asks the doctor to send a blood sample for testing. On a day when I visited, he had just received a message about a 340-pound 9-year-old. "The odds that there's something amiss there are extremely high," he said. "We will look at that child very, very carefully for variants in these genes and others . . . without necessarily anticipating that we'll be of any help to that child in the immediate sense."

🐾🐾🐾

Obese people today are living in a time that is both promising and painfully difficult. Although doctors have begun to recognize that body size is to a great degree determined by a person's genetic and biological vulnerability to weight gain and thus largely beyond an individual's conscious control, the science of obesity is still young. Despite the rapid pace of new discoveries in the field—and the wealth of scientific talent and pharmaceutical and government funding now focused on it—specific, highly effective treatments for obesity have yet to be discovered.

Meanwhile, we are facing an expanding public health crisis that clearly has not arisen because of newly mutated genes. Obesity is increasing at an unprecedented rate in the United States and in many other countries, and recent shifts in the environment are undoubtedly at the root of the epidemic. A "toxic environment," in the words of researcher Kelly Brownell of Yale University, is playing on individual genetic vulnerability to produce unhealthy weight gain in more and more people. And if environmental factors are at fault, then by changing the environment—or by learning ways in which we can consciously change our responses to it—it may be possible to slow down or even reverse the trend.

At a time when overweight people might be expected to take a measure of comfort in the recognition that their problem has a biological basis, society is delivering a confusing double message. Half of the message says: obesity is a disease, much like high blood pressure, and treatment should be covered by insurance. The solution, when it is discovered, will be a medical one. The other half says: for many people, unhealthy weight gain can probably be prevented if we can figure out which environmental factors contribute to it. Be more active, drink less soda, change your diet, and you can somehow escape it or ameliorate it.

How can this apparent contradiction be understood? And how can we, individually and as a society, work on preventing obesity—especially in our children—without continuing to make fat people feel, as they have for generations, that their weight problem must be all their fault? To answer the question we must explore scientists' current understanding of why so many children and adults are becoming overweight. Their genes may have established their individual risk of storing excess body fat, but factors in the environment are what make it happen.

The genes children inherit from their parents appear to be the strongest influence on whether they will become overweight, either in childhood or as adults. Some of the best scientific evidence supporting the hefty contribution of heredity comes from studies of identical twins and from studies of children who were adopted—the kind of research that has classically been used to tease apart the tangled influences of genes and environment on a host of conditions ranging from high blood pressure and colon cancer to various mental illnesses. In the case of obesity, although many studies suggest that genes are a bigger player than environmental factors, the modern environment may be shifting that balance somewhat.

For example, in 1990 psychiatrist Albert J. Stunkard of the University of Pennsylvania reported on 93 pairs of identical twins who had been raised in separate families and 154 pairs who had grown up together. The weight, height, and body shape of the identical twins separated at birth were astonishingly similar—almost as much alike as the weight, height, and bodies of twins who had grown up in the same family. Stunkard concluded that hereditary factors account for about 70 percent of obesity and environmental factors for only about 30 percent. Moreover, the study suggested that any impact of environment on obesity appeared to be derived from factors common to society at large, not from factors operating within the family.

In another study published in 1986, Stunkard and colleagues

looked at genetics versus family environment in a group of 540 Danish people who had been adopted as infants. Adult adoptees were categorized by "weight class": thin, medium, overweight, or obese. The weight class of the adult adoptees correlated with the BMIs of their biological parents (especially those of their mothers) and did not correlate at all with the BMIs of their adoptive mothers or fathers. Overweight adoptees tended to have overweight biological parents; lean ones tended to have lean parents. "Genetic influences have an important role in determining human fatness in adults," the research team concluded, "whereas the family environment alone has no apparent effect."

No apparent effect! The tone of these studies on twins and adoptees makes it seem as if it doesn't matter how parents feed their babies, what kind of snacks they provide, or whether they encourage their children to turn off the television and play outside. No matter what parents do, a child's weight and body shape will probably resemble the mother's or father's. "Adoption studies are the strongest evidence of there not being much influence of the family environment" on body size, says researcher Jane Wardle of the Health Behavior Unit at London's University College. Adopted children "remain as similar to their biological parents as [children who] were raised with their biological parents."

But not so fast. Not all studies have concluded that heredity predominates over environmental factors in determining who becomes overweight. In a recent review of about 50 studies of twins, adoptees, and nuclear families, researchers concluded that genes account for only about 25 to 40 percent of the variation in people's tendency to store excess body fat. Some researchers suggest that people can probably be categorized according to their degree of inherited risk: genetic obesity, strong genetic predisposition, slight genetic predisposition, and genetic resistance to becoming overweight.

One reason why studies have yielded such widely varying estimates of the role of heredity in obesity is that such estimates depend in part on the environment of the people being studied. If their environment is one that promotes weight gain, the role of genetic factors will appear smaller than if the environment is less obesigenic. Obesity is not unique in this respect. Many human characteristics—as well as many diseases—are the product of varying degrees of interaction between "nature" and "nurture." It's helpful to compare the evidence for heredity's role in obesity with the evidence for its role in some other conditions. For example, research indicates that the influence of genetics on body weight is as strong as its influence on height. Studies of twins tell us that genetics plays as great a role in establishing obesity risk as in the risk of developing schizophrenia, alcoholism, or high blood pressure.

But while it's true that a child's genetic endowment determines his or her vulnerability to weight gain, genes alone don't dictate what each individual's weight will be. If genes accounted for everything, the current epidemic of obesity would not be happening. Many aspects of our modern environment are undoubtedly contributing to that epidemic by encouraging people to eat more and to move around less. Environmental factors operating before birth and during infancy may also be influencing children's brain development and thus the ability of their bodies to regulate food intake. Parents—as well as other concerned adults—can affect how children handle their environment to some extent, by teaching good eating habits and by helping them be as active as possible. Nevertheless, researchers studying the epidemic believe that a comprehensive solution to the rise in obesity will require broad environmental and social changes.

Most of the modern world's impact on body size comes from our common, shared environment typified by the abundance of cheap, tasty, high-calorie foods; our reliance on cars, elevators, and other forms of motorized transportation; our sedentary lifestyle; and the difficulty of incorporating walking and other kinds of activity into our daily routines. To halt the obesity epidemic, we will have to identify which of these factors are most strongly contributing to weight gain and find ways to alter them—a daunting task.

The vast majority of children and adults who are overweight do not have a single defective gene as the cause of their weight problem. Instead, each has multiple genes that predispose that individual to eat a few extra calories, burn up less energy than they take in, or store the excess as fat. Like the members of a band, this collection of genes plays together to determine their possessor's vulnerability to putting on extra pounds. One person's band is not the same as another's: they may have some instruments in common and others they do not share. But each individual's combo of obesity-related genes plays along with various factors in the environment to determine that person's chances of becoming overweight.

How many genes might be at play? Researchers don't yet know. At one time many thought there must.be a single obesity gene—and when leptin was discovered, some believed at first that the master gene had been found. Now at least 60 genes are being investigated, and some scientists fear as many as 100 genes could be contributing to obesity risk. "One hundred genes, each with 1 percent effect," says Rudy Leibel. "Which from a genetic point of view is a nightmare."

Leibel's own suspicion, after examining patterns of obesity inheritance in families drawn from various populations and ethnic groups, is that the number of important players is much smaller. He suggests that each person may have up to a dozen genes that combine to determine individual obesity risk. Some of them—perhaps six or seven—are probably major players that help determine the likelihood of obesity in people all over the planet. The rest may be due to gene variants more common in one ethnic population than another, so that genes predisposing someone of Mexican descent to obesity might differ from those determining risk for Polynesians. "This is what makes the genetics so complicated," Leibel says. "We don't know which ones are the major players and we don't know which ones are the minor players. So we don't know how to apportion our efforts."

Although genes determine individual vulnerability to weight gain, environmental factors help dictate the outcome—the weight that a person reaches during childhood or adulthood. "What the genetics does is, it tells you, if you have 100 people, how they'll line up relative to each other in most environments," Leibel says. "It tells you, 'This is number 1 and this is number 100,' and how to rank people in between, in terms of body fat. What it doesn't tell you is what those 100 people are going to look like specifically in any given environment." For example, if 100 people were exposed to famine and had to subsist on a starvation diet, they would all become thin—but some would lose less weight than others. "Some of them are going to weigh 40 pounds and some of them are going to weigh 70, and this is going to be due to the genetics of how they dispose of the calories in the presence of severe calorie restriction," notes Leibel. "And the same is going to be true if you put them in fast food heaven. They're all going to get fatter, but they'll probably all get fatter in the same rank order."

Evidence of how tightly the body regulates its own energy balance is the fact that the majority of people do not become severely obese even in today's calorie-rich environment. The average person consumes 7.5 million to 10 million calories in the course of a decade, yet Americans and people in other Western countries typically gain only half a pound to a pound each year during their adult lives. In order to gain any weight at all, they must eat more calories than they burn— but the amount needed to account for this degree of weight gain is only about 10 to 20 calories per day, or about the equivalent of one Ritz cracker. That's less than 1 percent of an adult's average daily intake.

A calorie imbalance this small can't be reliably measured by researchers studying people in their normal habitat. To perform quantitative studies on how weight gain and loss affect people's appetite and metabolism, Leibel and his associates had to confine his volunteers in hospital research wards and measure every mouthful. He found, surprisingly, that obese people do not eat more than lean people in proportion to their body size. Of course, an obese person *does* have to consume a larger number of calories per day than a lean person of the same height simply to support a bigger body mass. But when allowances are made for the differences in body size, the number of calories consumed "per pound" is the same. Nor do obese individuals have slower metabolisms than lean ones, as long as they remain at the weight that is "normal" for them. They still balance their calorie intake and output very precisely to maintain a constant weight, just as lean people do. But the weight that they maintain is higher. Obesity "is a disorder which is the result of very, very small differences" in physiology, Leibel says. "You don't need a big error [in energy balance] to get a very big aggregate change in body mass over time."

The laws of thermodynamics dictate that people who are overweight must, at some point, have taken in more energy than they spent in order to gain the extra pounds. "There's no way around it," Leibel says. "You cannot eat like a canary and become the size of a pterodactyl." But in most cases, once obese people have reached a personal set point determined by their own physiology, their weight stabilizes. Their food intake and their metabolic rates, when adjusted for their body size, are similar to those of lean people.

However, when a person loses weight, the situation shifts dramatically. If lean or obese people lose 10 percent to 20 percent of their body weight, their bodies respond by becoming more efficient and using less energy in an effort to conserve calories and replenish the lost fat stores. This reduction in energy expenditure is much larger than would be expected for the amount of weight lost. "You see an adjustment of energy expenditure which is far greater—about 15 percent greater—than you would have predicted based on the change in body size," Leibel says. "This is big—and it accounts, almost certainly, for some of the tremendous recidivism to obesity that characterizes 90 to 95 percent of otherwise successful weight reduction." Studies suggest that about 95 percent of people who lose weight by dieting gain it back within five years.

In someone who has lost weight, resting metabolic rate drops. Muscles also become more efficient, so moving around and exercising burn up fewer calories than they did before the weight loss. There are shifts in hormone levels and in the fine-tuning of the nervous system that reduce energy consumption. In addition, even though the body is using fewer calories, people who have lost significant amounts of weight become uncomfortably hungry. Whether the amount lost was 10 percent of body weight, 20 percent, or even more doesn't seem to matter: the sensation of hunger is about the same, according to Leibel's studies. "It's very uncomfortable," he says. "Your body is essentially responding as if you were in a partly starved metabolic state." In many people who have lost weight, that sensation of increased hunger seems to persist, sometimes for years. Forced to fight such insistent signals from their own bodies, most people eventually regain the lost weight.

Leibel believes that, for adults, trying to keep weight off in the face of the body's determined effort to gain it back may be as difficult as trying to resist thirst or to consciously control blood pressure. Various studies indicate that regular exercise helps people maintain weight loss by burning calories and increasing metabolic rate. Yet exercise also unconsciously triggers increased food intake. That is why elite athletes in training do not spontaneously lose large amounts of weight: without having to think about it, they eat more to make up for what they burn. Many studies have found that by itself exercise doesn't produce much weight loss, although it definitely makes people fitter and healthier.

There is some evidence to support the theory that as a child goes through puberty, hormones and other biological influences act on the brain to establish what the permanent set point for body weight will be during adult life. Before puberty, the set point may not yet be firmly established, so loss of body fat may not trigger the same vigorous physiological responses in a child that it does in an adult. This biological difference may explain why some clinical studies have found that overweight children who have not yet entered puberty have higher success rates in losing and keeping off weight than adolescents or adults do. Such findings underscore the urgency of treating obese children as early as possible to help them achieve a healthier body weight.

The combination of genes each person inherits probably operates in various ways to determine individual vulnerability to obesity. "There are many people who have been dealt a hand that, in this environment, makes them become overweight," says Susan Z. Yanovski, a National Institutes of Health (NIH) official who is coordinating research on obesity prevention. Some genes, for example, endow those who carry them with a slower-than-average resting metabolism or a metabolic propensity to store calories as fat. Some genes may confer a taste for high-fat foods or a tendency to eat a larger quantity before feeling full than other people. Some make their possessors especially calm and sedentary, less likely than others to burn energy by fidgeting, moving around, or exercising.

Some of the most intriguing clues about how genes interact with the environment to make people fat come from studies in the Pima

Indians of southwestern Arizona. The Arizona Pimas have one of the highest rates of obesity in the world—rivaled only by the populations of a few western Pacific islands—as well as the highest reported prevalence of type 2 diabetes, a form of the disease that frequently develops in fat adults and is becoming increasingly common in overweight children. Surveyed in 1988 when the current national obesity epidemic was just getting under way, more than 80 percent of Pimas between the ages of 20 and 55 were overweight, and 40 to 70 percent were obese, with BMIs above 30. More than half of Pima adults over the age of 35 have diabetes.

For many years NIH researchers based at a government laboratory in Phoenix have been studying Pima volunteers from the nearby Gila River Indian Community to investigate why the Pimas' genes predispose them so strongly to weight gain. The Pimas, who call themselves Akimel O'odham (the River People), have lived in southwestern Arizona for at least 2,000 years. They practiced traditional methods of agriculture and farming until white settlers diverted the Gila River in the late nineteenth century. Today they eat a modern American diet, and many live on an arid reservation in the Sonoran Desert where snakes, packs of roving dogs, and extremely high temperatures make outdoor exercise dangerous.

For most of their history, the Pimas' traditional lifestyle as subsistence farmers in a harsh environment exposed them to periods of extreme privation and placed strenuous demands upon their bodies. Researcher James Neel proposed in the 1960s that such extreme environmental pressure on a human population might have favored the selective survival of individuals who carried a "thrifty gene," one that enabled them to store calories as fat during periods of plenty so they could live through periods of famine. Although the concept of a single thrifty gene has given way to the current "polygenic," or many-gene, theory of obesity, most researchers still agree with Neel's central idea, that a history of privation tends to make a population more vulnerable to weight gain and obesity. According to this theory, the extreme obesity seen in inhabitants of certain Pacific islands may occur because their ancestors frequently had to survive similar privation, perhaps during long inter-island canoe voyages.

In times of famine, "you would expect the fattest individuals to be the survivors," says Eric Ravussin of Louisiana's Pennington Biomedical Research Center, who spent 14 years studying the Pimas. "This gene pool has been protective for Pima Indians over their history." In a 1994 study Ravussin compared a group of Arizona Pimas with a group of Pimas who live in a remote mountainous region of northern Mexico. Although the Mexican Pimas speak the same language as members of the Arizona group, they are the descendants of people who separated from the Arizona Pimas about 1,000 years ago. They are physically active subsistence farmers, with a lifestyle similar to that of the Arizona Pimas' ancestors. Even though the two groups are thought to be closely genetically related, the Mexican Pimas are generally lean. In a comparison study that matched Mexican and Arizona Pimas by age and sex, Ravussin found that the Mexican Pimas weighed, on average, 57 pounds less than the Arizona Pimas. Their average BMI was 24.9 (within the normal range) versus 33.4 (obese) for the Arizona Pimas studied. Among the Mexican Pimas, the frequency of diabetes was 11 percent for women and 6 percent for men, compared with 37 percent among Arizona Pima women and 54 percent among Arizona Pima men at that time. These findings strongly suggest that it is the modern American diet and lifestyle, interacting with an obesity-prone genetic profile, that have made the Arizona Pimas suffer so severely from weight gain and its medical complications.

Just what is it about the Pimas' biology that predisposes them to weight gain? For many years, researchers thought the cause might be a slow resting metabolic rate or a tendency to store fat efficiently. But Ravussin and other researchers found that, on average, Pimas' resting metabolic rate, including that of the slender Mexican Pimas, was not significantly different from that of Caucasians. Certain characteristics did seem to run in families, such as a low metabolic rate or a physiological tendency to burn carbohydrates for energy in preference to fats. Fidgetiness—and the lack of it—also seemed to be inherited tendencies. But the research indicated that such traits explain only a little of the individual variation in obesity risk seen among Pima Indians.

A low rate of calorie burning does not appear to be at the root of the Pimas' inherited vulnerability to obesity. "Indirectly, through all this investigating of energy expenditure, we have kind of convinced ourselves that the main culprit must be a tendency to eat in excess of energy requirements," says Antonio Tataranni, the director of the NIH's Clinical Research Center in Phoenix. Rudy Leibel notes that studies of animal models of obesity, as well as studies of humans with monogenic obesity, tend to support that hypothesis. The evidence from those studies suggests that the most important contributor to the obesity is intake of excess calories, not a reduction in energy expenditure.

Most of the earlier studies on Pimas were performed with adult volunteers, but recently NIH researchers have begun to focus more attention on children. They have learned, for example, that excess weight gain in Pima youngsters may begin as early as the first month of life. In a 2002 study Robert S. Lindsay and colleagues reported that the pattern of weight gain in Pima children differs markedly from U.S. national norms, with Pima babies putting on significantly more weight for their length between the ages of 1 month and 6 months. Pima children between the ages of 2 and 11 also gain weight faster and have higher BMIs than national norms. Researchers are uncertain whether the rapid weight gain in infancy represents purely fat accumulation, nor do they know whether it's genetic or whether it's related to environmental factors during pregnancy or infancy. They are more confident that the rapid weight gain after age 2 reflects a tendency to gain fat. Current and future research will focus in greater detail on family eating habits and Pima children's food choices, Tataranni says.

Studies in these children, who belong to one of the most obesity-prone populations in the world, serve to underscore the importance of exercise. Pima children between the ages of 5 and 10 are four times more likely to be obese than children in the general U.S. population. Yet even among these children, being active and participating in sports do seem to help protect against both weight gain and the development of insulin resistance, a hormonal condition that is a precursor to diabetes. A 2002 study by Arline D. Salbe and colleagues found that Pima 5- and 10-year-olds who participated in more sports or recreational activities were less likely to be obese. Television had the opposite effect, just as many studies in children from other populations have found. Pima children's body weight and body fat went up in proportion to the number of hours of television they watched. Pima children who stayed active between the ages of 5 and 10 were less likely than others to gain large amounts of fat, and their bodies responded more normally to insulin, Tataranni and his researchers found. "Those kids who were able to maintain a more active lifestyle through these five years of observation did a little better," he says.

🐾🐾🐾

Rudy Leibel takes pride in the fact that his genetic research has served to shift blame for fatness away from the people who suffer from it. The ongoing discovery of obesity genes is proof that biological variations in vulnerability to weight gain are the major reason why some people are fat and others are lean. That's why Leibel views much of the current national debate about measures to prevent obesity with some concern. He points out that no one yet knows precisely what actions will be most effective. "On some level this is a disease that everybody thinks they understand, and yet in fact nobody understands," he says. "Everybody thinks they're an expert on this. They can tell you, 'It's the Coke in the schools. It's McDonald's.' Everybody has an explanation for it. But nobody really knows—including me and Randall and Randall's mother."

Seriously overweight people are doubly cursed: they have a dangerous medical condition that is notoriously resistant to treatment, and the rest of society makes them feel it must be their fault. "Most people who are 'experts' on obesity never really understood what it is like to have this problem," Leibel says. "It is a biological disorder that is attributed by everybody, including the patient, as being due to some failing that you can't identify. . . . It's a heavy burden to bear."

If everyone in the United States had the same genetic vulnerability to obesity, researchers could conduct a study to determine which environmental factors are most strongly influencing the epidemic. They could easily design trials to compare different strategies for preventing weight gain and learn which ones are most effective. Such a trial, for example, might be theoretically possible in the Pima Indians—who are more genetically homogeneous than the U.S. population as a whole—but it would still have to be a very large and long-lasting study.

Faced with the rapid rise of obesity in the U.S. population—and with the specter of accompanying increases in diabetes, heart disease, and other medical consequences—many researchers and public health officials are not willing to wait for the studies that could answer the question. They are designing and testing prevention programs for children that typically combine several strategies, such as education about healthy eating habits, physical activity sessions, and efforts to reduce television watching. Meanwhile, public and private campaigns are being launched at the local, state, and national levels to change Americans' diets and encourage them to exercise.

Leibel concedes that a lot of the advice seems like common sense. Some of the changes in behavior being promoted have other well-established benefits. For example, our population will be healthier in many ways if people can be persuaded to walk more, to breastfeed their infants, or to eat more fruits and vegetables. But as a scientist, he cautions that we should not assume either that the obesity epidemic has a single cause or that combating it will necessarily require draconian actions. "A relatively subtle intervention could have a big effect over time," he says. Yet because scientists can't measure either food intake or energy expenditure with enough precision in people living normal lives outside a hospital research laboratory, they can't quantify the relative contributions of excess calories and insufficient physical activity to the obesity epidemic, much less pinpoint the precise roles of many of the "usual suspects," such as soda and fast food consumption or a reduction in the amount of time children spend playing outside. "We really don't know what has happened, other than on a very macro, thermodynamic level," Leibel says. "Food intake is greater than energy expenditure. Period."

CHAPTER 3

Size, Health, and Self-Esteem

The girls of the Bold and Beautiful Club are on the move. In sneakers, sweatpants, and T-shirts or tank tops, they burst out the doors of Walker Upper Elementary School into the warm spring afternoon. There's Marcie, a broad-shouldered, wisecracking girl in a bright yellow top. There's Brianna, quiet and bespectacled with pigtails. There's JaNia, a cheery, talkative girl with straightened black hair, and her giggly walking partner Noelle, whose precise braids frame her head. Eight girls—tall ones and short ones, African Americans and whites—set off up briskly up a hill with two female guidance counselors on an after-school walk in suburban Charlottesville, Virginia. What these girls have in common is the reason they were invited to join this club: they are all what they prefer to call "big."

Their bodies fill—and in many cases strain—the fabric of their pants and tops. They are fifth- and sixth-graders, aged 10 to 13, but some are already physically developed and could be mistaken for high school students. Walking uphill in the sunshine is difficult for most of them. They puff and sweat as they march along, some girls swaying with every step as they throw one ample leg slightly out to the side to ease it past the other. Each set of partners has been given the same list of things to look for—a red bird, a flower, a female jogger, a parked blue car, a small child playing, evidence of roadkill—and they eagerly scan the streets and lawns, shouting as they spot an item on the list to check off.

For its members, the Bold and Beautiful Club meetings on Monday afternoons are a high point of the week. Each session starts with some exercise—walking, dancing, aerobics—and then moves on to a lesson on nutrition or personal health and hygiene. There's usually a healthy snack that the girls eat and learn how to make at home. And there are special attractions: guest speakers, field trips, swimming parties, sessions on skin care or makeup. "It's a lot of fun," confides JaNia. "There's a lot of activities, and I like it."

Halfway through the walk, nobody has spotted a red bird, roadkill, or a runner. "If you want to check off a female jogger, you have to do a little jogging yourself," says Minda Barnett, a counselor who is the club's coleader. Nobody takes her up on that suggestion, but the girls do pick up their pace as they start down a steep slope. Marcie throws herself to the ground and lies supine on the pavement. "Here's your roadkill," she says. Everyone laughs. By the time they reach the bottom they're getting hot and tired. The pair in the lead spots a child playing in a park at the end of a lane; the panting stragglers try to get away with checking off that item without going to look. "Oh, no," chides Barnett. "You have to go up there and see the kid."

Back in their classroom, club members drink lots of water and eat "ants on a log" (celery spread with low-fat cream cheese and sprinkled with raisins or sunflower seeds). Miss Lamb, a science teacher, arrives with creams, lotions, washcloths, and makeup mirrors to teach them how to give themselves a facial. She passes out the supplies and talks about skin care. The girls set up the magnifying mirrors and peer at their faces intently.

"What do you see?" asks Miss Lamb.

"I see bumps," says Ashley, a girl with braids and big dark eyes.

"I got dry skin," says someone else.

Miss Lamb shows them how to apply a cleanser and moisturizing cream. For the next few minutes the room is all but silent as the girls concentrate on making small circles with their fingers, rubbing in cream until their cheeks and foreheads are shiny. Suddenly they're children again, giggling and playing peekaboo with the mirrors.

"Raise your hand so I know you're listening," says Miss Lamb. "What have you learned from this today?"

"Not to use bar soap," says JaNia.

"What if you did this every day?" asks Miss Lamb.

"Oh, you'd be beautiful," sighs Ashley.

Like many communities in the United States, Charlottesville has a burgeoning epidemic of childhood obesity: a 2001 survey of third-grade students in the town's public schools found that almost 42 percent had BMIs above the 85th percentile for their age, meaning that they were already either overweight or at risk of becoming so. The Bold and Beautiful Club is so named for good reason. Barnett founded it about seven years ago for fifth- and sixth-grade girls who were overweight and, in the opinion of their teachers or counselors, had low self-esteem. With help from local nutritionists, Barnett and fellow guidance counselor Atalaya Sergi developed an after-school program aimed at making club members feel better about themselves, fostering friendships with other girls, and encouraging them to adopt healthier eating habits and increase their physical activity. A comparable program for overweight boys has also been offered at the school, but this year Barnett could not find any male teachers or counselors to lead it. Similar school-based programs for overweight children have been implemented around the country. Such programs provide vulnerable children with needed social support and may increase the likelihood that they will adopt healthier habits, although so far there has been little formal evidence that they prevent or reduce obesity. In the Charlottesville program, the goal is improving girls' self-esteem and promoting healthy behavior, not producing weight loss; girls are not weighed at the sessions, and dieting is not encouraged. Since no study has been conducted to compare BMI changes among Bold and Beautiful members with those in a similar group of nonparticipating girls, it's impossible to determine whether the program reduces girls' obesity risk.

For children of both sexes, but especially for girls, being overweight can be a daunting social and emotional burden. In the idiom of mainstream American culture, fat is considered unattractive. In films, television, advertising, and other media, the dominant images of physical beauty are inextricably linked with slenderness: thin thighs, wasp waists, muscular arms and buttocks. This societal obsession with thinness is pervasive and infectious: studies reveal that even in the early elementary grades, many girls begin to fret about their body shape and say they want to lose weight. In a survey by Stanford University researchers of more than 900 California third-grade students, 35 percent of white girls, 44 percent of Latinas, 28 percent of Asian American and 50 percent of African American girls said they wanted to lose weight. Among Latina and Asian American girls, studies suggest that the desire to be thin is every bit as strong as among white girls. In African American culture, large women have traditionally been considered attractive and sexually desirable, a shared value that has helped protect overweight African American girls from some of the distress suffered by heavy girls of other racial or ethnic groups. Among white girls, higher socioeconomic status and higher levels of education are associated with lower levels of obesity; those patterns have not consistently been found among African American girls. But there is some research evidence, such as the Stanford study mentioned above, that the media-driven taste for thinness also influences the self-image and eating habits of African American girls.

The girls of Bold and Beautiful are clearly vulnerable to such influences. Outside Barnett and Sergi's office hangs a poster made by club members, a collage showing glamorous African American and white models. Almost all are willowy, long-legged women wearing sexy, revealing fashions. Other photos depict short skirts, elaborate hairstyles, and handsome, well-muscled men. Only one image shows a voluptuous large woman, her legs hidden beneath a long full skirt. Barnett said club members made the poster after being instructed to look through women's magazines and find images of women they thought were beautiful. After they had assembled the collage, the counselors told them about the techniques used by photographers to touch up and modify images, and they discussed the high incidence of eating disorders among young female models. Then they asked the girls to peruse the magazines again, this time searching for a picture of someone who looked like a real person. "Many of the girls said they couldn't find anyone who looked real to them," Barnett recalled.

On the day I visited, I received an impromptu lesson about how easily a discussion of children's body size can slip into the territory of value judgments and self-esteem. The girls asked me what my book was about. I explained that more and more children in our country are becoming "big" and that bigness is a problem because carrying extra weight is not healthy for kids. When I told them I didn't yet have a title, they piped up with suggestions.

"The Bad Behavior Story," offered Ashley.

I said I didn't think being overweight meant that a person was "bad."

Casey, another student, came up with an alternative. "How about Big People, Small World?"

Helping overweight children without adding to the shame and stigma many of them already feel is a challenge that confronts parents, doctors, and anyone else who works with kids. In the past, fear of causing children psychological distress, fear of making them weight obsessed, and even fear of triggering an eating disorder have sometimes prevented doctors from trying to treat children's obesity. "It's like the emperor with no clothes," says Nazrat Mirza, a pediatrician at Children's National Medical Center, in Washington, D.C. "Obesity has been gradually increasing. Somehow we've really turned a blind eye to it.... The epidemic is here and we haven't done anything."

A vibrant and idealistic doctor who earlier in her career treated malnutrition among the Masai in her native Kenya, Mirza was stunned, on moving to the United States, at how many of her young American patients were overweight. She says that often, when she begins to counsel parents about an overweight youngster, they tell her she is the first doctor who has ever mentioned that their child has a weight problem. "Nobody addresses it," she says. "They are afraid to tip the scale into eating disorders. I'm not saying that's not something we should be sensitive to, but I don't see why we shouldn't address the obesity. Obesity kills."

Conversely, Nancy McLaren, a clinical associate professor of pediatrics and medical director of the Teen Health Center at the University of Virginia, in Charlottesville, says she believes that most pediatricians today are fully aware of the obesity epidemic and are attempting to grapple with the problem. "There's so much more in the medical literature and so much more at conferences—and there's much more on the news," she says. "They are trying to take a more proactive role with it."

Mirza says that, in the past, she has heard pediatricians worry that raising concerns about overweight could cause a vulnerable child to develop an eating disorder. The most dreaded one is anorexia nervosa, a rare but life-threatening condition that most often affects white teenage girls. Anorexia nervosa, estimated to affect between 0.5 percent and 3.7 percent of women during their lifetime, is commonest during adolescence, and appears to be especially rare in African American girls. Its relative frequency in other racial or ethnic groups is uncertain. A girl with anorexia nervosa obsessively reduces her food intake to lose weight, and may remain convinced that she is fat even when she has become dangerously emaciated and ill. A somewhat commoner eating disorder, bulimia nervosa (estimated to affect between 1.1 percent and 4.2 percent of females sometime in their lives), is characterized by deliberate, repeated, and often secret vomiting or laxative use to prevent weight gain, often after episodes of binge eating. Both of these conditions can cause serious, even fatal, medical complications—but so can obesity, which is far more widespread among children in the United States, where almost one-third of our nation's children are obese or are considered medically at risk of becoming so.

Binge eating disorder is a third, more frequent condition that can coexist with and contribute to obesity, although most overweight children and adults are not binge eaters. During any given six-month period, between 2 percent and 5 percent of Americans are thought to experience binge eating disorder. Symptoms include frequent, recurrent episodes of overeating associated with feelings of guilt and loss of control—but not accompanied by unhealthy compensatory measures like self-induced vomiting or laxative use.

"The relationship between eating disorders and obesity is a complex one," notes Susan Yanovski, an obesity expert at the NIH's National Institute of Diabetes and Digestive and Kidney Diseases. "For example, obesity is a risk factor for the development of eating disorders, but there are also data suggesting that disordered eating may play a role in the development of obesity in susceptible individuals."

Pediatric obesity experts emphasize that there is no evidence that a sensitive effort by a doctor to treat an overweight child increases the risk of triggering an eating disorder. On the contrary, some studies suggest that teaching healthier eating habits to obese children and their families may actually reduce the incidence of eating disorders.

There are other reasons why many doctors may be reluctant to confront the problem of overweight kids. Getting into the issue with families is delicate and time-consuming; it's a sensitive subject requiring tact, a detailed discussion about the child's and family's eating habits and activity levels, and plenty of parent education. The doctor needs to teach parents strategies to address the child's weight problem other than "putting the child on a diet," a frequent parental response that, as I will explain, can be counterproductive and even harmful. It is virtually impossible to pack all of the necessary questions and information into a "well-child" visit, which typically is a 15- or 20-minute annual checkup that includes a physical examination, immunizations, and brief counseling about a variety of other topics. And obesity in children or adults currently is not a "reimbursable diagnosis," as Mirza points out: insurance typically does not cover the cost of separate visits to a doctor or dietitian for treatment—until obesity has become severe enough to cause a medical illness. That may change in the future, because government officials recently asked federal Medicare administrators to gather evidence on whether particular treatments for obesity are effective and should be covered by the plan. If Medicare begins to cover obesity treatment, other insurers are likely to follow.

In addition, physicians have traditionally received little nutrition education or training in how to assess a growing child's caloric needs and how to counsel the mother or father of an obese patient. "They don't know what to do," Mirza says. "We say, 'Refer the patient to the nutritionist.'" But because of the demands on nutritionists' time at her hospital, she notes, "If I refer to the nutritionist today, they might be seen in two months or three months."

Considering these disincentives, it is little wonder that doctors and other health care providers often do not address excess weight adequately in children and may not even record it as a problem in the medical record. A 2002 study found that the medical evaluation of overweight children and adolescents fell far short of nationally recommended practice guidelines. Fewer than 10 percent of practitioners answering a national survey followed all the guidelines when taking a medical history and examining overweight children. A majority did not routinely perform recommended checks for bone and joint abnormalities, sleep disorders, or impaired glucose metabolism that could signal impending diabetes, all serious problems that can develop in obese kids. "Oftentimes a pediatrician sees a child who is overweight and then you wonder, OK, do I really want to go into the spiel of the disease complications?" Mirza says. "Obesity is a chronic problem and there's a lot of work involved. Most providers would say they're unsuccessful [in treating it]. There's this feeling of futility."

Defining "overweight" in children is more difficult than in adults, because a child's body mass index, or BMI—the ratio of weight to the square of height—changes as the child grows. BMI normally goes down during early childhood (until around the age of 5 or 6), because during this period boys' and girls' height is increasing faster than their weight. Through the rest of childhood and early adolescence, BMI rises steadily as children grow taller and put on weight. In both sexes, BMI continues to increase throughout the teenage years, though somewhat more gradually for girls than for boys.

BMI does not correlate perfectly with fatness, because changes in body mass reflect changes in both fat and muscle. Thus, for example, an athlete with a large muscle mass could have a relatively high BMI but very low body fat. Accurately measuring body fat stores is too complicated and expensive to use as a screening method for identifying those who are overweight, so BMI has been adopted as a surrogate measure that correlates reasonably well with fatness for most people. If a child has a high BMI and there is uncertainty about whether the measurement reflects excess body fat or muscle mass, a doctor or other health care professional can easily check by using calipers to measure skin-fold thicknesses at various points on the body, which is another way to assess fat stores.

Parents are not necessarily good judges of whether or not their children are carrying too much body fat. In a study of more than 600 mothers of preschoolers (aged 2 to 5), Amy E. Baughcum and colleagues found that 79 percent of the mothers with overweight children failed to perceive their kids as overweight. (They were somewhat more realistic about their own body size: 95 percent of obese mothers accurately believed that they were overweight, but one-third of normal-weight women also thought of themselves as too heavy!)

A larger national study that included a wider age range—5,500 children between the ages of 2 and 11—found that nearly one-third of mothers whose children were overweight failed to correctly classify their children as overweight. A mother's race or ethnicity had no impact on how likely she was to misjudge her child's weight status. The study also exposed an interesting difference when it came to gender. Girls whose BMI placed them in the "at risk of overweight" category were almost three times more likely than boys in that same group to be judged "overweight" by their mothers. That finding suggests that mothers may hold daughters to a stricter body size standard than sons, perhaps because of the cultural emphasis on female slenderness. "Mothers' negative perceptions of their daughter's weight status may contribute to young girls being extraordinarily pressured to engage in weight control practices," the authors commented.

Making parents aware of the health risks for children of being overweight—and getting them to act when a child is gaining too much weight—is the focus of a policy issued in 2003 by the American Academy of Pediatrics (AAP). It recommends that doctors should measure and chart BMI at least once a year in all children and adolescents. It also urges doctors to identify and track young patients at special risk of becoming overweight because of a family history of obesity, an unusually high birth weight, or various socioeconomic, ethnic, cultural, or environmental factors. And it recommends that doctors watch for too-rapid changes in BMI (signaling that a child's weight is climbing faster than expected) to identify those children at risk of becoming overweight and take early preventive action.

"By age 5, if your child is significantly overweight, you're already on the path to disease outcomes," says Deborah Young-Hyman, a clinical psychologist and obesity researcher at the NIH's National Institute of Child Health and Human Development. "There seems to be a disconnect, currently, between parental understanding of overweight and its health risks that potentially is a new hook for pediatricians to start engaging parents in intervention."

Following the policy will require pediatricians to change their behavior. Pediatrician Nazrat Mirza notes that doctors have traditionally been trained to react quickly when a growth chart shows that a child is failing to gain weight as expected, a condition medically known as failure to thrive. "All the alarm bells begin to sound," she says. "We start getting really aggressive." In contrast, when a growth chart shows that a child's BMI is climbing upward, crossing percentile lines (a much commoner situation among kids in the United States today), "no alarm bells sound," Mirza points out.

It's a good idea for parents to ask their pediatrician to provide them with a copy of the standard growth chart used in children's medical records so they too can keep track of their child's height and weight at the time of each annual physical (and at other medical visits, if they are measured then). Current growth charts also show the range of normal BMIs for age and sex, so parents can take the chart along to appointments and ask the pediatrician to mark the child's BMI on the graph.

Some school districts, concerned about the pediatric obesity epidemic, have decided not to rely on doctors to alert parents whose children are overweight. Instead, they're sending home health and fitness report cards—nicknamed "fat letters" by some critics—to encourage families to instill healthier habits. At least one state—Arkansas—is in the process of adopting such a program statewide. A study of one such effort in Cambridge, Massachusetts, found that among parents who received such letters, 42 percent of those with overweight kids reported efforts to boost their children's physical activity, 25 percent said they would consult the child's doctor, and 19 percent said they planned to put the child on a diet. Among parents of overweight kids who did not receive such reports, only 13 percent reported plans to take any of those measures.

The Cambridge study also suggests one of the pitfalls of informing parents that they have an overweight child without giving them much guidance about what to do next. The study's authors were pleased about parents planning to encourage physical activity or consulting their child's pediatrician but were upset that almost one-fifth said they intended to try to control their child's weight through dieting. Educational materials sent home with the reports had urged families to limit children's TV time to no more than two hours per day, to encourage an hour a day of physical activity, and to try to make sure that children got at least 5 daily servings of fruits and vegetables. These materials also specifically discouraged parents from trying to place their overweight child on a restrictive diet, an approach that various studies have shown can actually be counterproductive. Medically unsupervised, do-it-yourself weight-loss diets are not a safe or healthy option for children and adolescents, and efforts by a parent to tightly control a child's food intake are likely to backfire. A recent three-year study by researchers at Harvard Medical School found that girls and boys who were frequent dieters gained more weight annually than those who never dieted and were also more likely to become binge eaters. Dieting has become such a common behavior pattern in our society that many parents apparently assumed it was the right approach.

Sherry Arria, mother of an overweight 10-year-old, described to a *New York Times* reporter the mixed emotions she felt on receiving one of those "fat letters" from the Cambridge Health Department. Diabetic since childhood, Arria had grown up craving all the foods she wasn't allowed. Now she found herself locked in a food struggle with her daughter. "If I walk out of the kitchen, she'll jump up and eat food real quick," Arria said. "I hate that. I don't want to run back to catch her, because I don't want her to feel bad about it. . . . I don't want my daughter to be obsessed with her weight. Briana's weight has even been an issue with my family. They hate the fact that Briana is heavy and try to pin it on me. . . . Meanwhile, I'm struggling to figure it out myself."

Parents do need to monitor their children's eating patterns, but those who focus obsessively and critically on a child's weight or eating may do considerable harm. Some research suggests that too-tight parental control over a child's food choices and intake may be counterproductive, working against children's innate ability to monitor their own hunger or satiety. Such findings are an important reason why experts advise parents not to respond to a child who seems to be gaining too much weight by "putting the child on a diet."

Nutrition researchers Leann L. Birch, Susan L. Johnson, and Jennifer O. Fisher have done extensive studies on how parenting affects young children's ability to adjust how much they eat in response to their hunger level and to the calorie density of food. In a 1994 laboratory study of 77 boys and girls between the ages of 3 and 5, Johnson and Birch found that the very children whose mothers tried hardest to control how much they ate were the ones least able to regulate their own intake.

Birch and Fisher have also periodically studied a group of 140 Pennsylvania girls and their parents, recording the children's weight and height, and gathering information and experimental data when the girls were 5, 7, and 9 years old. They classified the girls according to whether they were overweight or lean and also according to the level of restriction (high or low) mothers exerted over their food choices and intake. At each of the three ages they also performed a laboratory experiment in which the girls were fed an ample lunch and were then given access to a variety of tasty snacks during a brief play session. The researchers measured how much of the available snacks the children (who all reported after lunch that they were not hungry) ate. They found that "eating in the absence of hunger," as measured by the after-lunch snacking, increased for the entire group between the ages of 5 and 9, suggesting that children's eating becomes more influenced by cues from the environment as they get older. However, eating in the absence of hunger increased more among those girls whose mothers had used higher levels of food restriction when they were 5 years old. Girls who had been overweight at 5 and whose mothers had also highly restricted their food intake showed the greatest degree of overeating at the age of 9.

In related studies, Birch and Fisher reported that young children whose mothers restricted their eating were more likely than other children to be overweight. They also found that mothers who had a personal history of dieting and unhealthy weight gain tended to try to exert more control over their daughters' intake. The researchers suggest that such early dietary restriction may predispose girls, at least, to develop a variety of unhealthy eating patterns. Such findings are controversial. Birch and Fisher have mainly studied middle-class white girls, and they emphasize that their provocative conclusion—that parental dietary restriction may impair girls' ability to regulate their own food intake—might not apply to boys or to other races and ethnic groups. Indeed, some other scientists have failed to replicate their findings. Stanford researchers studied almost 800 third-graders from diverse ethnic and socioeconomic backgrounds and concluded that girls whose parents controlled their food intake tended to be *less* overweight, not more so.

Birch and Fisher's findings do not answer the question of whether too much parental control over a child's food intake can actually cause the child to overeat, or whether it is the child's innate or genetic propensity to overeat that has triggered the parents' control efforts, notes William H. Dietz, an expert on pediatric obesity at the federal Centers for Disease Control and Prevention. "Are these parents who are controlling children's intake because they already know [the children] can't control themselves, or is lack of control on the part of the child a consequence [of the parents' approach]?" he asks. To answer that question, he added, researchers would need longitudinal studies that would follow children over a longer period of time. "I think she [Birch] has shown, at least to my satisfaction, that parents who control their children's intake have children who are less capable of doing so themselves," Dietz says. "I think that this kind of parenting affects food choices. But it may not affect weight long term."

Attempts by researchers to investigate whether parental feeding styles can contribute to childhood obesity "generally show very inconsistent results," notes Jane Wardle, a professor of clinical psychology at London's University College. Some studies suggest that the strongest parental efforts to control children's eating occur not when a child is overweight but when a parent perceives a child as underweight and "neophobic"—unwilling to try new or unfamiliar foods. Wardle notes that at a well-regarded pediatric obesity treatment program at Great

Ormond Street Hospital, in London, a study found that parents of overweight children entering the program were relatively unlikely to have tried to control their children's diets prior to the start of treatment. During treatment, however, they became more likely to monitor intake and to prompt their children to eat healthy foods. At the same time, the parents of children being treated also became less likely to use food as a reward or as an all-purpose remedy for emotional distress.

Those findings underscore a point made consistently by experts in childhood obesity: effective strategies for changing eating behavior should involve teaching the entire family, not just the overweight child, new habits.

🐾🐾🐾

How bad does a child feel about being fat? Does being overweight cause depression in children? Conversely, can being depressed cause obesity? Although hundreds of studies have been done to explore such topics, there are no simple answers. The short answer to all three of those questions appears to be: it depends.

Children and adults become overweight because some combination of environmental influences interacts with their body's genetic propensity to store fat. But once a child is overweight, the way those excess pounds affect how that child feels about himself or herself depends on many factors, including the child's age, sex, and personality; the child's relationships with family members; the response of friends and peers; the child's racial or ethnic group; and the social and cultural environment. "One assumes that obesity is detrimental to children's psychological adaptation, and it just isn't necessarily so," says psychologist Deborah Young-Hyman. "It depends on a whole constellation of things."

Children's self-esteem depends on how they assess their abilities in a variety of areas—whether they feel smart, strong, and capable, whether they can make and keep friends, whether they feel loved and valued, as well as how they feel about their bodies. For toddlers and young children, much of that self-assessment reflects the feedback they get from parents, siblings, and others in their immediate family. Once children enter school, the responses of others their age begin to influence the picture—and become increasingly important as they get older, especially in adolescence. School-age kids and adolescents are also highly influenced by positive and negative feedback from other powerful adults in their lives, such as teachers, coaches, doctors, and members of their extended families.

Modern American culture teaches children to stigmatize those who are fat. In a study conducted in 2001 of several hundred fifth- and sixth-grade students, Rutgers researchers asked participants to rank six drawings of children—including one showing an obese child, several showing children with disabilities, and one of a child who was thin and not disabled—according to how well they "liked" each child. The students ranked the drawing of the slender child without disability highest and the drawing of the obese child lowest. Compared with results of a similar study performed in 1961, the difference in "liking" between the top-ranked nondisabled child and the obese child was about 40 percent greater in 2001, suggesting that stigmatization of overweight children has worsened in recent decades, despite the fact that such children have become far more numerous.

Because overweight children tend to be taller than their peers, adults often assume they are older than they are and may subject them to unrealistic expectations. It's not entirely clear why most overweight children are also taller than average, but their rapid growth in height may be due to the effects of elevated levels of insulin and related circulating "growth factors," combined with an abundance of building material in the form of nutrients. In girls, high levels of body fat are also associated with hormonal alterations that often lead to an earlier-than-average onset of puberty, with accompanying body changes that can provoke or intensify teasing by other kids.

Discrimination may continue into young adulthood, especially for women. One study found that overweight girls, even though equally academically qualified, were less likely to gain acceptance to elite colleges than their slender peers. A large government-funded study, the National Longitudinal Survey of Youth, found that women who were obese in late adolescence and young adulthood achieved lower levels of education, had lower incomes, had higher rates of poverty, and were less likely to marry than peers who were not overweight.

In a study entitled "Are Overweight Children Unhappy?" a team of researchers measured weights and heights of more than 800 third-grade students in northern California public schools and asked the children to complete questionnaires about body weight concerns and symptoms of depression. They found evidence that high BMIs correlated with depression in the girls but not in the boys. Those girls who expressed concern about their weight were also most likely to report symptoms of depression.

In other studies of northern California students, Stanford University researcher Tom Robinson and colleagues found that by the age of 8, worries about weight and body dissatisfaction are common among both girls and boys, regardless of ethnic group or socioeconomic status. Among white, Hispanic, and Asian girls in the sixth and seventh grades, Robinson found, body size (as measured by BMI) was the strongest predictor of body dissatisfaction. But in a group of more than 100 overweight African American children living in Baltimore, Deborah Young-Hyman could find no significant impact of weight on the children's overall self-esteem, even though many of the children in the study (who ranged in age from 5 to 10) were very obese. Among children 8 or older, those who were very overweight did have more negative feelings about their appearance, as did those children whose parents considered them overweight. These findings may reflect the fact that in African American communities large body size is more culturally acceptable than among other racial and ethnic groups in the United States.

A key point identified in Young-Hyman's study and in several others is the importance of weight-related teasing as a cause of psychological damage in overweight children. In her study, the fattest children reported more frequent peer teasing and less social acceptance. Those children were also most likely to have fought with others because of their weight, using aggression to defend themselves from teasing but, as a result, often getting into trouble with their parents and teachers. Young-Hyman notes that aggressive behavior may have helped these children preserve their self-esteem.

Among adolescents, teasing and social stigmatization of fat kids seem to be more severe than among younger children, and the consequences are especially troubling. For both boys and girls in middle school and high school, regardless of race or ethnic group, being teased about weight is linked with low self-esteem, symptoms of depression, thoughts of suicide, and even suicide attempts. In a study of more than 4,700 students in grades 7 through 12, Marla E. Eisenberg of the University of Minnesota found that it was the teasing, rather than the children's actual weight, that predicted depression and suicide risk. Teasing was particularly hurtful when it came not just from peers but also from a child's family. For example, Eisenberg found that almost one-quarter of adolescent girls teased about their weight by both peers and family members reported that they had attempted suicide, compared with about 8 percent of adolescent girls who had not been teased. Among both boys and girls, those who had suffered weight-related teasing (whether for being overweight or underweight) were two to three times more likely to consider or attempt suicide than those who had not.

Overweight adolescents tend to have fewer friends than lean children do, according to a national study that surveyed more than 90,000 middle and high school students about how many people they considered to be their friends. Overweight children were almost twice as likely as lean children not to be named as a friend by any other child. Tracey Saxon, a teacher in Charlottesville, says she sees the damaging effects of teasing and social isolation on some of the overweight sixth-graders she teaches. "I think that their body images right now vary," she says. "If they have friends and are accepted, they're kind of indifferent. If they have been picked on, then they're very upset. They have very low self-esteem. And that carries over, obviously, to the classroom."

At the urging of researcher Michael Rich, a few overweight Boston-area teenagers have captured on video some of the personal pain hidden behind the scientific findings. Rich, an adolescent medicine specialist at Boston's Children's Hospital, gave some of his young obese patients a camcorder and asked them to record their lives or their thoughts, creating what he calls a visual illness narrative. He asked his subjects' permission to study the videotapes and to use them as a tool for teaching doctors, health care workers, and others who work with children about the psychological impact of obesity. Some kids talked directly to the camera; some set it up as a silent spectator as they went through their days. "The camcorder sort of functions as a confessional," Rich says. "They show things to the camcorder that they are not able to share with the physician."

In one clip, a heavyset girl wearing a red kerchief tells the camera, "I think sometimes the reason why I eat the way I eat is because I'm either mad or I'm sad or people look at me strange. . . . It's like I'll eat even if I'm not hungry. If I'm hurting, sometimes that's when I eat the most." In another, a dark-haired, overweight boy stares impassively into space while his father, sitting nearby, criticizes him: "Lazy—lack of direction—lack of ambition. . . ."

In another sequence, a fat boy rants about Leonardo DiCaprio. "He sucks! He just has to shake his hair back [to get a girl], and we have to work so hard to get a date." A curly-haired, obese girl tells the camera defiantly, "I like myself the way I am! On the other hand, if you want to lose the weight, do it for yourself and do it because you want to and not because other people are forcing you, not because of the pressures of society. . . . I could have lost the weight five years ago, but I never did because it was like me saying, 'F— you' to the whole world. I don't have to conform to your images."

Despite the social isolation and criticism many overweight kids endure, studies suggest that the majority of overweight children and adolescents are not clinically depressed. Depression in children, however, is a serious and underrecognized problem that should be identified and treated whenever present. An illness in its own right, it carries a risk of suicide. Some research suggests that it also increases the likelihood that a normal-weight child will become overweight and that an already overweight one will continue to gain.

A key study sheds helpful light on the chicken-and-egg question about whether being fat is a risk factor for becoming depressed or vice versa. Researchers Elizabeth Goodman and Robert C. Whitaker performed a prospective study of more than 9,000 children in grades 7 through 12 who were interviewed at home on two different occasions, one year apart, for a large government-funded survey of adolescent health. Overweight adolescents were no more likely to be depressed than lean ones, according to the results of the baseline interview. (Of the total sample, 8.8 percent were depressed, as measured by a questionnaire that assesses depressive symptoms. Among the obese children, 8.2 percent were depressed, compared with 8.9 percent of the non-obese ones.) Surprisingly, the results indicated that being fat did not increase a child's risk of developing depression over time either. At the follow-up interview a year later, children who had been obese at baseline had the same frequency of depression as children who had been lean.

But a depressed child or teenager, whether fat or lean, *is* at risk of gaining unhealthy amounts of weight, the study showed. Children who had been depressed at the baseline interview were significantly more likely to be obese a year later, compared with those who had not been depressed. Among kids who were already obese at the baseline interview, those who were also depressed gained more weight during the follow-up year than those who were not. Goodman and Whitaker suggest that there may be a subgroup of children or adolescents who respond to depression by developing an increased appetite or binge eating episodes; treating the depression effectively might prevent such individuals from developing obesity. There is also evidence from other research that depression or chronic stress can lead to persistently high levels of cortisol, a hormone that promotes weight gain as well as abdominal fat deposition and some of the other features of the metabolic syndrome. Such findings are a powerful argument for paying attention to children's emotional well-being as an important influence on their physical health.

Some children also gain unhealthy amounts of weight as a response to physical or sexual abuse or emotional neglect. Doctors should ask questions that can help identify such factors when evaluating a child who is gaining too much weight.

Leonard H. Epstein, director of a nationally known treatment program for overweight children in Buffalo, New York, says he often sees cases in which depression or other psychological problems, such as binge eating disorder, developed before a child became heavy but were ignored or left untreated. "Parents, a lot of times, think, 'If my child was just thin, the depression would go away,'" Epstein says.

When it comes to a child's body size and self-esteem, there are many factors that parents simply can't control. They can't do anything about their genetic inheritance, which may include a propensity to gain weight that they have passed along to their offspring. They can't completely shield their children, whether fat or lean, from exposure to the unhealthy aspects of modern society, from being influenced by the opinions or behavior of their peers, or even from hurtful teasing. They may not be able to prevent their child from becoming overweight or from suffering some of the physical and psychological consequences of carrying excess body fat.

But there is much that parents and other caring adults can do to raise children who are self-confident and resilient, who value themselves and other people for who they are on the inside and not just for what they look like on the outside. Adults impart such qualities and values as much by their own, often unconscious, behavior and attitudes as by what they say. Talking with a child who may be developing a weight problem, teaching a child about why healthy eating and exercise habits are important, will be far easier if that child feels loved and valued by the person who is doing the talking. And listening—paying attention to children's feelings and opinions, finding out about their friendships and interactions with others—is just as important as talking, perhaps more so.

Parenting is a complicated job, one that human beings do not instinctively know how to do. It takes years—and plenty of help and guidance from others—to become an expert. Nevertheless, a number of valuable lessons and strategies have been developed by people who have worked with families in research and treatment settings. They have found that parents can learn to use language, styles of interacting, and positive reinforcement to maximize the likelihood that their kids will adopt healthier habits—by choice, not under duress.

Learning to accentuate the positive is vital, states Epstein. He believes that his treatment program for overweight kids owes its high long-term success rates to its focus on teaching highly effective parenting techniques and using behavior therapy to change the habits of the entire family. He urges parents to use praise, not blame or criticism, to influence their kids. "One of the things I've been most surprised about is how hard it is for parents to generalize" this principle, he says. "When we teach them to praise kids for eating healthier, you would think they would start thinking, 'I can use praise, then, for other behaviors.' They don't. They don't generalize."

Children are acutely sensitive to criticism by parents and other family members, even though they may not show it and may even seem to shrug it off. Marla Eisenberg's study dramatically showed how overweight adolescents suffer when teased about their weight by others in their families. Charlottesville teacher Tracey Saxon says her former sixth-graders would sometimes tell her that their normal-weight parents were "disgusted" with them for being fat—and she has seen how badly children are hurt by such attitudes. NIH researcher Sue Yanovski says she tells parents of overweight children, "Your kids know that they're fat. You don't have to constantly remind them of it. You need to let them know you love them regardless of size."

Whether trying to prevent children from becoming overweight or helping those who are already too heavy, adults must teach kids the benefits of choosing healthy foods, watching their portion sizes, and staying active, and they should model those habits. They should emphasize that the most important reason for adults and children to try to avoid becoming too heavy is that it is bad for their bodies. If an overweight child needs treatment, parents should address this with the child as a medical problem, not as a matter of physical appearance or as a focus for blame.

Leonard Epstein and his staff teach parents how to positively reinforce the behaviors and habits they want to encourage in their children, rather than constantly criticizing kids for things they do wrong. He said such a shift makes children feel as if they are the ones in control. "It makes a tremendous difference in the way kids approach things," he says. "Say a parent wants to get the child to do their homework. The parent recognizes that one of the things that competes with doing homework is TV. Most parents would say, 'You can't watch TV until you finish your homework.'" But a parent using positive reinforcement would say, "After you finish your homework, then you can watch TV," Epstein adds. "It's a huge difference in the [child's] perception of what the parent is trying to do."

As part of Epstein's program, parents and children agree on goals—such as reducing the number of hours a child watches TV and substituting some form of physical activity. They also agree on rewards the child can earn by achieving the goals. The rewards must not be food or things that cost money, such as toys. Instead, they are usually privileges or activities the child and parent agree to do together. Epstein's research suggests that a vital ingredient in the success of his program is that the child is given choices. For instance, children can choose the kind of activity they want to do, and when they are hungry, they can choose a snack from a variety of healthy foods. Allowing some choice "is just critical," Epstein says. "I think that's what good therapists do: they get people to do what they want them to do, but make it appear as if it's their choice. If it's your choice, you buy into it. If you are doing it just because somebody told you to do it, it doesn't necessarily make you buy into it."

This doesn't mean that a child's choices should be limitless. William Dietz of the CDC emphasizes the importance of teaching children that the evening's dinner menu is whatever a parent has prepared. Parents shouldn't get into protracted negotiations with children who refuse what is served, Dietz believes. "Parents need to set limits on that. It's OK for a parent to say, 'If you ask me one more time, you're going to have to take a time-out.' They need to be able to buffer themselves from these kinds of incessant requests or complaints."

Consistency is key, which means double standards within families don't work either. Children will see them as unfair and will quickly rebel. For example, parents cannot expect to drink soda or eat doughnuts at home but forbid a child to have those items. In addition, they should not forbid an overweight child to have candy or potato chips while allowing the child's normal-weight siblings to eat them. "It creates second-class citizenship for the child in the home," says psychologist Young-Hyman. Rather than being food policemen, Epstein suggests, "Rearrange the environment. Give the child the choice of 2, 5, 10, or 15 healthy things" as snacks, and make the same choices available to everyone in the household.

Children can and should be included in family discussions about why parents choose to offer certain foods at home and not others.

"Have candid discussions with kids," says David L. Katz of the Yale University School of Medicine's Prevention Research Center. "Say, 'Look, in our family we are going to balance eating the things that taste really good with the importance of eating things for our health. We'll make compromises, but we're going to pay attention to the way we eat to make sure we protect ourselves.' That way, nobody is being disciplined, nobody is being punished or made to feel bad."

Food should never be used as a bribe or as a reward, nor should restricting or forbidding food ever be used to punish a child. One aspect of teaching children how to recognize and respond to their own internal signals of hunger and satiety is to try to separate food, as much as possible, from some of the other ways in which it has come to be used in our society. We all grow up in cultures where food has traditional roles and meanings. Our lives would be impoverished if all of those meanings were removed. Yet to fight the obesity epidemic that threatens our children's health, we must identify some of the societal and cultural reasons why adults and children eat more than they need, and we must be willing to change those patterns. We may have to abandon habits learned in childhood or revise our beloved but unhealthy family recipes.

"Eating is how most of our cultures evolved," notes pediatrician Nazrat Mirza. "We celebrate birth with eating. We celebrate death with eating. You tell your kids, 'OK, you've been so good, let's go to McDonald's.' It's kind of all wrong. We really have to change our way of thinking about how we're going to reward children. We have to show them that, yes, we can celebrate without food."

🐾🐾🐾

Just as we, as a society, must change some of the ways we use food, so we must also work to shift cultural perceptions so that obesity is recognized as a threat to health, not a cosmetic problem. Tracey Saxon embodies that distinction for the girls of the Bold and Beautiful Club. She is 36 years old, overweight, and diabetic. Not long ago she weighed 350 pounds. "You are the person you are because of a lot of things," Saxon says she tells the club members. "Weight is one of them. It's nothing to be ashamed of."

The daughter of a high school football coach, Saxon was a gifted athlete who played Division I field hockey and lacrosse in college. She was always overweight—but she was physically active, outgoing, and had plenty of friends. "I was proud to be big and strong," she recalls. She grew up feeling great about her body. "My mom is close to 6 feet tall and overweight," she confides. "My dad says every day that she's the most beautiful woman in the world." She says she promised herself, however, that if her size ever caused health problems or prevented her from doing something she wanted to do, she would try to lose some of the excess pounds. That day arrived a couple of years ago when her doctor discovered that she had diabetes. He warned her that she could lose her feet or her eyesight if she did not lose weight. She cut back on potatoes, bread, and other carbohydrates. She joined a gym and began working out daily. Over a period of months she lost 70 pounds and brought her diabetes under control. "My goal out of this is not weight loss," she says. "I want to be healthy. My doctors say they think that healthy for me is going to be around 200 pounds. With my body type and the way I'm built, that may be perfect for me. . . . Healthy comes in different numbers."

Although Saxon says she feels well, having diabetes has changed her life. She wishes she had learned earlier that the disease runs in her family. "One of the things I tell the girls is, talk to your parents," she says. "Ask them questions. Heredity plays a major role, especially if your family has a history of obesity."

"I've had to learn a lot about food and how to do these crazy [calorie] counts," she adds. "It's a pain for me. I tell the girls, if you can learn to make just a couple of better choices a day, you'll never get to this point. . . . My big thing that I try to tell them is, it doesn't matter what you look like as long as you're healthy. As long as you can live the life you want to live."

CHAPTER 4

Teaching Children
How to Eat for Life

Nine-year-old Adam has learned a new way to eat—and so have the other members of his family. Fried potato chips have been banished from the kitchen shelves in Adam's home in Newton, a leafy Boston suburb. French fries are not on the family menu either. Pizza, when it's served, is often homemade on small loaves of whole wheat pita bread. All of these staples of the modern American diet used to be among Adam's favorites, but he eats them now only as an occasional treat.

For breakfast on a recent morning, Adam—a friendly, articulate boy with striking gray-green eyes—had a bowl of high-fiber cereal with milk and a big bowl of mixed fruit: grapes, blueberries, melon, strawberries, and cantaloupe. On other days he eats a cooked egg white with low-fat cheese on an English muffin, or lox and light cream cheese on half a bagel. The lunch he carries to school typically includes a peanut butter sandwich, fruit, yogurt, and skim milk. He often snacks on high-fiber, low-fat health bars or cucumber pickles—and he drinks plenty of water. Adam does not consider his new pattern of food choices a "diet." He calls it an eating plan, or a healthier way to eat. When I visited Adam's home one spring afternoon, he had been following it for almost a year. His parents and his 5-year-old sister were eating according to the plan, too. "I've been doing really well on it, and I'm going to keep it up," he said.

Adam learned about the eating plan at Optimum Weight for Life, or OWL, a research and treatment program for overweight children directed by David Ludwig, a Harvard pediatrician and obesity researcher at Boston's Children's Hospital. OWL is based on a growing body of research by Ludwig and others suggesting that a diet rich in fruits and vegetables but low in refined starches and sugars, and which also contains protein, unprocessed whole grains, some dairy products, and a moderate amount of fat, may be healthy for the heart and least conducive to weight gain and diabetes. In the medical literature, such an eating plan is called a low-glycemic-index diet.

Adam's mother, Laura, knew by the time her son was 8 that he would need to learn to manage his weight. As an adult, she had experienced her own weight problems and had joined Weight Watchers to revise her eating habits. Adam's father had also struggled intermittently with weight gain. At 8, Adam was big for his age and, as his mother put it, "a good eater"—in fact, he seemed to be hungry all the time. A picture taken that summer shows a round-faced, chubby child. The family's pediatrician, concerned that the boy was unhealthily heavy, referred Adam to OWL, which treats overweight kids 4 and older. After Adam underwent an initial medical evaluation, he and his parents attended group sessions to learn about the new eating plan. He returned to the OWL clinic for follow-up visits about every two months.

Adam remembers watching a slide show that taught him the basics of the plan while his parents learned how it is thought to work. Starchy foods like potatoes or bread made from white flour are rapidly broken down to sugar by the body, tending to raise blood sugar levels rapidly and trigger a corresponding surge in insulin. A few fruits—bananas and watermelon, for instance—also cause a quick surge in blood sugar. Such foods are said to have a high glycemic index. ("Glycemic" is a medical term that means "putting sugar into the blood.") On the other hand, protein and fat, as well as most fruits and vegetables, which are high in fiber, take longer to digest so they raise blood sugar more gradually and do not provoke such a large or sudden insulin surge. Hence, they have a low glycemic index.

Whole grains that have not undergone much grinding or processing are also digested slowly, but the same whole grain can turn into a food with a high glycemic index if it has been finely milled. (For example, highly processed "instant" oatmeal has a high glycemic index, while relatively intact, slow-cooking "steel-cut" oatmeal has a low one.) In addition, including some fat as part of a meal slows the emptying of the stomach, so that nutrients are not delivered too rapidly to the intestines, where digestion and absorption into the bloodstream take place. Studies by Ludwig and his research team have found that children who were given a breakfast containing foods with a low glycemic index were less hungry during the day, and consumed fewer calories, than those who ate a breakfast containing an equal number of calories but composed of high-glycemic-index foods.

To Laura, part of the appeal of the OWL program was that its research suggested that while following the plan Adam would be less eager for snacks between meals—although healthy snacks are permitted in moderation. The insulin surge triggered by foods with a high glycemic index produces a corresponding plunge in the blood sugar level a few hours later. When blood sugar drops too low, there is a compensatory rise in other hormones, including the "stress" hormones epinephrine and cortisol, and hunger kicks in. In Ludwig's studies, children and adults given low-glycemic-index diets have smaller ups and downs in blood sugar and lower insulin levels than those following a conventional low-fat diet, and they report less hunger. Laura also liked the plan's flexibility. "What I think works about it is, it doesn't say 'You can't have' and 'You can have,'" she observes. "It tries to say 'More of this, less of that.' You keep foods in proportion."

Following the plan required big changes in Adam's eating habits. His family had always eaten salad or vegetables with dinner, but Adam loved junk food, his mother says. Potatoes, especially French fries, were also a particular favorite, but they have an especially high glycemic index. "At the start, it was just so hard for me," Adam recalls. At one point "I said, 'I can't do this,' and I almost stopped. But my mom and dad encouraged me to go back [to the plan] again." A year into the plan, Adam says he has gotten used to it and no longer finds it difficult to follow. "It's one of the easiest things I do," he remarks. "It's just part of my regular schedule. I don't sneak treats at school or anything."

The family's shopping and cooking habits have also changed. They eat many more fruits and vegetables. Laura often grills or broils fish and, if she fries food, she uses olive oil. She routinely packs lunches at home rather than allow her children to buy lunch at school. She limits calories and fat in the family pantry by buying low-calorie bread, lean meats, and light margarine. She also invents recipes. "She made up a new fajita that's yummy," Adam says proudly.

For Adam's family, switching to the plan wasn't easy. Adam's little sister is a picky eater and sometimes complains about missing the snack foods her mother no longer buys. "Our food bills are high," says Laura. "To eat healthy is very expensive." She estimates that she spends $100 more each week at the grocery store than her friends do, but also notes that she does save money by making three lunches a day instead of paying for them at school or work.

The results have been worth it. At 9, Adam looks like a different child. He weighs 34 pounds less now than he did last year, even though he's been growing. He is slender and muscular. "I'm faster. I'm just much stronger now," he says. He joined a swim team at the Newton YMCA and won a medal in the winter at the district championships. In the spring he joined a baseball team. Says Laura, "I think one of the reasons Adam never liked soccer was that it was too hard. He had trouble keeping up with the kids. Now he can. He can do what everybody else does."

Adam still visits the OWL clinic for periodic checkups. "I'm not exactly trying to lose weight," he says. "I'm just trying to stay on the plan and keep going." According to his mother, "He knows what he can eat and what he can't eat. It works for him. I really feel that if he learns that now, it's a lesson that he can take through his life and always come back to."

🐾🐾🐾

Following a low-glycemic-index eating plan like the one taught at the Boston OWL clinic is not the single "right" way for a child or a family to learn to eat healthily. In fact, despite the popularity of weight-loss regimens such as the South Beach Diet that are founded on similar concepts, most nutrition experts concur that diets based on foods' glycemic index still need additional study, especially in large clinical trials designed to test their long-term effects on body weight and overall health. Nevertheless, the OWL plan's emphasis on eating plenty of fresh fruits and vegetables, whole grains, and nonfat or low-fat dairy products while including sources of "healthy" fats such as olive oil, nuts, and fish are principles that most nutrition scientists and dietitians heartily endorse. Most American families could probably benefit from some of the lessons about healthy eating that Adam and his family have learned.

In today's environment, parents can no longer take for granted that their children will grow up knowing how to make good food choices and maintain a desirable weight. The pervasive changes in our daily patterns of eating and activity make excess weight gain likely for just about everyone, at least at some time. Simply following one's urges regarding food and exercise probably will not work for most people. Teaching children to make choices that add up to a healthy lifestyle requires a degree of sophistication that simply was not necessary for parents in the past. "If the environment were not the way it is, it probably wouldn't matter if people had good parenting skills around food and physical activity," notes Shiriki K. Kumanyika, a professor of epidemiology at the University of Pennsylvania School of Medicine. But today's kids are far more sedentary than children were in past decades, and they live in an environment replete with high-calorie, tasty, heavily advertised food and drink. "We need to reeducate parents," Kumanyika says. "As a nutritionist, when I look at what people think they should feed their kids, they haven't a clue."

Parents have a limited number of influential years in which to teach their children good eating habits and instill attitudes about exercise and lifestyle that their offspring will need all their lives. Although many experts believe that major environmental changes would be the most effective way to reverse the obesity epidemic in the United States and elsewhere, no one is optimistic that such changes will happen rapidly—and they may not happen at all. In the meantime, one way to prevent obesity is to make parents more effective at "immunizing" their children against unhealthy weight gain. "It is not likely that we will ever return the environment to one in which . . . cognitive control of body weight is not required," predicts researcher James O. Hill, director of the University of Colorado's Center for Human Nutrition, in a recent article. "We should consider how to make sure that everyone has the information and tools needed to cognitively maintain energy balance."

A few striking statistics help to sketch a portrait of the calorie-laden dietary environment that is pushing Americans' weight steadily up the scale. The amount of food available to the U.S. population increased by 15 percent between 1970 and 1994, from 3,300 calories per person per day to 3,800. These figures don't mean Americans are eating that whopping number of daily calories, since they include food that spoils, is wasted, or is discarded, but they do show that our country's farms and food manufacturers are producing and marketing more food and drink than ever before—and they suggest that people have probably increased their caloric intake in response. A recent national survey indicates that American adults are indeed eating more than in the past. In the years 1999 and 2000, women were eating an average of 335 calories more per day than they ate during the early 1970s, and men were eating an average of 168 more calories per day. (The average daily caloric intake for women in 1999–2000 was 1,877 calories; for men, it was 2,618 calories.) These counts are based on 24-hour dietary recall data gathered from a national sample of people aged 20 to 74, as part of the government's periodic National Health and Nutrition Examination Surveys (NHANES), a series of large national studies conducted by the U.S. Department of Health and Human Services.

Obtaining accurate information about what people eat can be difficult, because people tend to underreport their intake or even lie about it, and many survey participants understandably have difficulty remembering every item on the previous day's menu. As a result, surveys by different government agencies sometimes obtain conflicting results. For example, in consecutive surveys by the U.S. Department of Agriculture (USDA), respondents reported consuming 7 percent fewer calories, on average, in 1994 than in 1978, and dietary data from the 1987 and 1992 National Health Interview Surveys also showed a modest decline in reported intake. However, the NHANES have consistently documented a gradual but steady increase in adults' reported intake over the past three decades. These findings, combined with data on food production and other evidence from a variety of smaller studies, point toward the conclusion that Americans are consuming more calories.

Among U.S. children the findings of various surveys tell a more consistent story: they show that children's average daily food intake has increased during the past quarter-century and even climbed slightly between the early and mid-1990s. Although underreporting of intake can affect the accuracy of data in children just as it can in adults, these cross-sectional studies—"snapshots" of dietary intake at different points in time— do suggest that today's children are eating more calories now than a decade or two ago.

Where are those calories coming from? Again, information from survey participants about what Americans are eating may appear, at first glance, to be at odds with food production figures. Consider fat intake. Population surveys show that Americans reduced their fat intake between 1970 and 1994, from 42 percent of daily calories down to 38 percent. They may have done so partly in response to federal dietary guidelines issued in the early 1990s, which recommended that total fat should make up no more than 30 percent of the diet and saturated fat no more than 10 percent. Yet fat production per capita in the United States actually increased during that period, again suggesting that the survey findings might not accurately reflect everything people eat. An intriguing possible explanation for these seemingly contradictory findings is that even though fat makes up a lower *percentage* of the average person's diet today than in 1970, American adults and children are eating more total calories—so their absolute daily intake of fat has actually risen. One analysis of children's intake concluded that although fat as a percentage of kids' diet fell from 38 percent to 32 percent between the early 1970s and the late 1990s, the actual amount of fat the average child eats each day has not declined because today's children are eating more calories than the children of three decades ago.

Today's children and adults drink far less milk than Americans did in past decades. Per capita milk consumption fell from 31 gallons in 1970 to 24 gallons by 1997. Milk consumption decreased by 37 percent in adolescent boys and by 30 percent in adolescent girls between the mid-1970s and the mid-1990s. Over the same period, soft drink consumption rose more dramatically than any other food category, suggesting that soda was replacing milk in the diets of many children and adults. By 1997 Americans were drinking 44.4 gallons of soft drinks per person per year, 10 gallons per person more than in 1987. Some children in the United States are introduced to soda before they reach their first birthday. By the age of 14, one-third of girls and more than half of boys are drinking three or more 8-ounce servings of soft drinks per day. This huge increase in soft drink consumption has helped boost Americans' intake of added sugars to about double the maximum level recommended by federal dietary guidelines. Added sugars, especially from soft drinks, currently make up 16 percent of Americans' total calorie intake—and 20 percent of the calorie intake of adolescents. Fructose, a major sweetener in soft drinks—and in many other products—is a sugar that does not trigger the same hormonal responses in the body as glucose, although it is chemically similar and contains the same number of calories per gram. Some experts have suggested that its increasing use in food and drink products since 1970 (when it was first marketed in the form of a sweetener called high-fructose corn syrup) may have played a role in the genesis of the obesity epidemic.

There is some evidence that high soft drink consumption may reduce children's intake of important nutrients from other sources, including calcium, phosphorus, and various vitamins. Epidemiological research in children has linked soft drink consumption with higher total daily calorie intake and increased risk of obesity. Those findings apply not just to sodas but also to fruit drinks that contain a small percentage of fruit juice diluted by a large volume of sugary water. Researchers conducting the Nurses' Health Study, a large, ongoing epidemiological study of U.S. women, recently reported that women who increased their consumption of sugar-sweetened soft drinks or fruit punch (from less than one drink a week to one or more drinks a day) gained significantly more weight over a four-year period than women who held their intake constant or reduced it. The same study also showed that high intake of sugar-sweetened soft drinks or fruit punch (consuming one such drink or more per day) is associated with an increased risk of diabetes, compared with the risk seen in women who consume such drinks infrequently (less than one drink per month).

Not all dairy consumption is down. As milk fell, cheese rose. Between 1970 and 1997 annual cheese consumption increased from 11 to 28 pounds per capita. Much of that increase may have been propelled by an explosion in the popularity of pizza, a food high in total and saturated fat whose consumption increased 150 percent between 1977 and 1994. Pizza, along with pasta, soft drinks, and Mexican food, also has contributed to the rise in children's daily calorie intake from carbohydrates—sugars and starches—during the past two decades. (Carbohydrates, fat, and protein as dietary calorie sources are discussed in detail later in this chapter.)

Meanwhile, Americans' intake of fruits and vegetables has risen since 1970 but not to the minimum levels recommended by the government's dietary guidelines, despite a federally financed advertising campaign to boost intake. In 1996 Americans ate an average of 1.3 servings of fruit per day, compared with 2 to 4 servings recommended in the guidelines, and they ate 3.8 servings of vegetables, compared with the recommended 3 to 5 servings. (According to the guidelines, examples of a serving are a single piece of fruit, 1 cup of raw leafy vegetables, or half a cup of chopped or cooked vegetables.) National dietary survey data collected between 1994 and 1996 reveal that children ate an average of 4.1 servings of fruits and vegetables daily, compared with the 5 recommended. Although these figures don't seem too far off-target, the picture is less encouraging when intake is examined in more detail. Children's average fruit intake, 1.4 servings per day, is below the minimum 2 servings per day recommended. French fried potatoes account for 46 percent of vegetable servings for children between the ages of 2 and 19, according to government data collected in 1999–2000. If potatoes were removed from the "vegetable" category, as some nutrition experts have advocated, children's vegetable intake would be much farther below the recommended target level. In contrast, dark green and orange vegetables, which are especially rich in vitamins, made up only 8 percent of kids' vegetable intake.

Indeed, despite the wide variety of fresh produce available in the United States, Americans of all ages tend to limit their consumption to just a few types. In 2000, five vegetables—iceberg lettuce, frozen potatoes, fresh potatoes, potato chips, and canned tomatoes—made up almost half of total vegetable servings, while orange juice, bananas, apple juice, apples, grapes, and watermelon accounted for half of all fruit servings.

Moreover, recent decades have seen a dramatic change in where our meals come from. A shift away from preparing food at home has been a major contributor to many of the alterations in the average American's diet, affecting not only the sources of calories but, perhaps even more important, the "portion size," or amount of a food or drink a person consumes during a meal or snack. This shift results from a variety of social and economic factors, including the high proportion of women who work, the growing complexity of family schedules, and the time demands of food shopping and cooking. Consumption of meals and snacks at fast food restaurants tripled between 1977 and 1995. By 1998, 21 percent of American households ate some form of take-out or delivered food on any given day. In 1997 nearly half of family expenditures for food were spent on food and drink prepared outside the home, and more than one-third were for fast food. By the mid-1990s, consumption of foods prepared away from home made up almost a third of children's total calorie intake. Both take-out and restaurant food tend to be higher in fat and calories than food cooked at home. Studies in teenagers and adults link frequent consumption of fast food with higher daily calorie intakes and higher body weights. A recent study found that teenagers served a fast food lunch ate an average of 1,652 calories during that single meal, more than 60 percent of their estimated daily energy requirement! Although all the kids in the study tended to overconsume fast food, overweight teens ate more than lean ones and were less likely to compensate by eating less at other meals during the day.

In addition, foods are being sold in increasingly larger portion sizes, a trend that has been under way for decades. A "portion" and a "serving" are not the same thing. A serving is a standard amount used to advise people about how much to eat or to specify the calorie and nutrient content of different foods. For example, in the federal government's dietary guidelines and Food Guide Pyramid, a serving of bread is a single slice and a serving of milk or yogurt is 1 cup. A portion, in contrast, is the amount of food placed on the plate or dispensed in a single-use container. The heaping portion of spaghetti customers often eat in Italian restaurants might amount to 4, 5, 6, or more pasta servings (defined as a half cup of cooked pasta). The recent expansion in the nation's portion sizes started as a marketing strategy by food manufacturers and the restaurant industry, but there is evidence that over time it has transformed Americans' cooking and eating behavior at home.

The amazing growth of the Coca-Cola container is a good illustration of the "supersizing" marketing trend. A bottle of Coca-Cola in 1916 held 6.5 ounces. By 1950, 10- and 12-ounce "king-sized" bottles were on the market, but the 6.5-ounce bottle was still the best-seller. Today, a regular can of Coca-Cola holds 12 ounces, 20-ounce bottles have become standard in many vending machines, and 32-ounce bottles are widely sold. Similar supersizing trends have occurred for fast food sandwiches, burgers, portions of French fries, bagels, popcorn, candy, and other products. The ballooning of portion sizes is reflected on grocery store shelves and even in cookbook recipes; researchers have documented it in almost every food category.

The hefty sizes are popular with consumers, who figure that larger-volume products are a better deal, and they are profitable for producers. But supersizing food portions trains people to overconsume. Often, the fine print on government-required food labels reveals that a bottle of sweetened fruit drink or a bag of chips contains several servings, yet the packaging and advertising for supersized products are designed to encourage the purchaser to eat or drink the whole thing. Research suggests that the supersizing of food portions adversely affects people's unconscious decisions about how much food to consume at one time and is directly correlated with Americans' increased calorie intake. In a fascinating series of studies involving foods as varied as chips, submarine sandwiches, and baked pasta, nutrition researcher Barbara J. Rolls of Pennsylvania State University has shown that the larger the portion, the more people eat—even though fewer than half of participants report noticing differences in the portion sizes they are served.

To find out whether young children respond in the same way, Rolls and her colleagues conducted a study in which children were served varying amounts of macaroni and cheese. The researchers found that 3-year-old children tended to eat the same amount regardless of portion size, but 5-year-olds ate larger amounts when given larger portions—suggesting that as children grow older, they become responsive to environmental cues that tend to override their body's internal satiety signals. In another study of preschool children, Rolls and colleagues found that when they doubled the size of an entree served at lunch, children increased the average size of each bite they took and as a result ate 25 percent more of it.

Prominent among the environmental stimuli that influence food choices and intake is ubiquitous food advertising. Food manufacturers, retailers, and services are second only to the automobile industry in money spent on advertising. Food and beverage advertisers spend an estimated $10 billion to $12 billion annually to promote their products to children and adolescents. A report released by the Kaiser Family Foundation in 2004 found that the typical American child sees about 40,000 advertisements per year on television and that the majority of TV ads targeting children are for candy, soda, and fast food. One study found that television commercials influence the food preferences of children as young as 3 to 5 years old.

In the U.S. population as a whole, foods that are most heavily advertised (snacks, candies, convenience foods, soft drinks, alcoholic beverages) are overconsumed relative to what is recommended in national dietary guidelines, while the least advertised foods, such as fruits and vegetables, are underconsumed. Although the U.S. Department of Agriculture spent about $1 million in 1999 to promote its "5 A Day" message encouraging people to eat more fruits and vegetables, the majority of Americans consume less. By comparison, McDonald's spent almost $572 million and Burger King $407 million on advertising in 1998.

"The entire culture has moved, in my view, in a direction that seems to be the worst direction if you're concerned about developing obesity," says researcher Michael Schwartz of the University of Washington. "If you wanted to see what is the environment that would maximize the rate of weight gain—we've more or less created it."

Faced with an environment packed with tasty, fattening foods and resounding with cues urging us to eat more of them, what can parents and other adults do to teach children to resist these seemingly irresistible forces? The good news is that, on an individual or a family level, the changes in behavior required to avoid weight gain may be less drastic than one might expect. Simply by making small changes in daily routines and in the home environment, parents have more power than they may think to improve the family diet and move their own habits and those of their children in a direction that can help everyone to achieve or maintain a healthy weight. University of Colorado's James Hill estimates that the "energy gap" causing so many children and adults to gradually gain weight probably amounts to an average of 100 calories per day—that is, on average, people are likely consuming about 100 calories more than they expend in activity. That's equivalent to about one slice of bread or two-thirds of a can of soda. Since excess caloric intake is stored with only about 50 percent efficiency, such an imbalance in energy intake would lead to about 50 extra calories being stored as fat—enough to account for the average weight gain of about 2 pounds per year seen in U.S. adults between the ages of 20 and 40.

It should be possible for many people to eat 100 fewer calories a day without drastically altering their lifestyle, Hill suggests. For instance, eating three bites less of a typical fast food hamburger could reduce intake by 100 calories. Moderately increasing daily activity would also help to close the gap, probably at least preventing further weight gain. Walking an extra mile each day, about 2,000 to 2,500 extra steps, would burn 100 calories. Because children do not inherently know how to make such choices, Hill writes, "as a society, we should be more willing . . . to carefully manage the food and physical activity environments of our children at home, in school, and in other places."

A diet high in fat and highly processed carbohydrates is probably the kind most likely to promote weight gain, yet this is the way most Americans eat, notes Michael Schwartz. He believes that parents can do a lot to prevent obesity in children by teaching them to be aware of their food choices and to make physical activity a habit. "As a parent, my personal feeling is, if people were as conditioned to exercise every day as they are to brush their teeth, I think that would go a long way," he says. In time, changes that start with individuals and families might lead to a shift in the norms of an entire society.

❧❧❧

People often complain about what they view as conflicting dietary advice from experts and inconsistent findings from scientific studies about nutrition, yet in many broad areas there is little or no disagreement. Experts on nutrition and obesity are virtually unanimous about a number of steps parents and other adults can take to improve the chances that the children they love will grow up with healthy eating habits.

As often as possible, meals should be a family activity, a time for parents and children to be together. Starting in infancy (discussed in Chapter 6), children should be able to see the face of the person feeding them. Just as a baby should never be put to bed with a bottle or propped in a seat with one, older children should generally not be expected to eat meals alone. It's also wise to limit eating and drinking to areas of the home such as the kitchen or dining room, since children become conditioned to expect food in physical settings where it is usually offered. In particular, parents should not allow children to eat—even snacks—while watching television. As I explain in the next chapter, there is ample research evidence that television viewing contributes in multiple ways to the epidemic of childhood obesity, and one of those ways is a tendency for kids to ingest excess calories almost unconsciously while watching TV.

Children generally do best with regularly scheduled meals each day—especially breakfast, which has been shown to improve their thinking skills as well as academic and physical performance. Recent studies in children and adults have also found that those who eat breakfast regularly are less likely to be overweight. It also appears that there is nothing magic about a three-meals-a-day schedule: one study found that adults who ate frequent small meals (four or more daily) were less likely to be obese than people who ate three large ones.

In addition to regular meals, many children, especially preschoolers and fast-growing adolescents, need snacks. However, significantly more U.S. children report consuming snacks today than in the 1970s, and this increased snacking has probably contributed to the rise in kids' calorie intake. Steering kids toward snacks that are not calorie dense, such as fresh fruits, vegetables, and nonfat or low-fat dairy products, can improve their diets and help limit excessive caloric intake.

Meals and snacks should not be rushed; eating at a leisurely pace allows time for the digestive tract and the brain to sense satiety and signal that it's time to stop. Some research on infants suggests that very rapid intake of calories is associated with excess weight gain and may lead to increased obesity risk. Slower ingestion of calories may be one reason why breast-fed babies have a lower risk of later obesity than bottle-fed ones. Eating out or picking up a take-out dinner is a convenience that few families will want to forgo entirely, but parents and others concerned about preventing obesity should resist the societal trend toward relying ever more heavily on restaurant or take-out food. A study of children and older adolescents found that those who ate dinner at home with their families consumed fewer fried foods (both at home and elsewhere) and less soda, and ate more fruits and vegetables, than those who did not.

Preparing a meal at home allows those who cook it to control the kinds of fats used (if any), the sugar and salt content, and whether foods are steamed, baked, boiled, grilled, or fried. It is difficult and sometimes impossible for consumers to influence what goes into a meal cooked in a restaurant or into a frozen entree or heat-and-serve item from the deli or supermarket. Sharing meal preparation with children also teaches them lifelong lessons about how to choose healthy foods and how to handle food safely, as well as imparting cooking skills and family and cultural traditions.

Although eating with the family is good for kids, highly charged emotional struggles focusing on food are not. Research has shown that absolute bans on certain foods are likely, paradoxically, to make children crave them more: telling a child "no French fries" is a surefire strategy for making them a favorite. Conversely, insisting that a child eat broccoli may trigger a fixed opposition to that vegetable. Parents can have a more positive impact by letting the child see them eating and enjoying the food they wish to promote (such as a cooked vegetable) and by encouraging the child to try a taste, even a tiny one, each time it is served. It's normal and expected for young children to distrust or reject an unfamiliar food, and research has shown that it may take 5 to 10 experiences with a new item before some children accept it. "Absolutely, repeated introductions do help a child get used to foods," says William Dietz of the CDC. "I think it's reasonable to suggest to a child that they have a bite of something."

Sheila Crye teaches after-school and summertime cooking classes to children between the ages of 9 and 14 at her home in a Washington, D.C., suburb. The parents of some of her students complain that their kids have been picky eaters all their lives. One boy wanted to become a chef but was unwilling to try the new dishes he was learning to make. "He'd look at something and he wouldn't even want to taste it," Crye recalls.

In an older child such reluctance may occasionally stem from an early unpleasant experience with a bad-tasting medicine or from a parent's ill-advised practice of putting peppery sauce on a child's tongue as a punishment ("saucing"). But many kids are simply cautious by nature and are slow to accept things that look, smell, and taste unfamiliar. Crye persuades her students to promise to taste what they cook. She tries to provide fresh ingredients whenever possible, believing that they make foods taste best. "It's a trust relationship," she says. She promises her students, "I'm going to help you fix things that you will like. I'm not going to make you eat anything really nasty." Because picky eaters will sometimes try to avoid tasting a new food by swallowing a bite as quickly as possible, she asks them to describe the flavor: "Is it salty? Is it sweet? Can you tell what spices are in it?" Crye tells parents: "Keep serving things that are normal, good foods. Make them take a taste. You don't have to fight about it. If you can get a commitment from them that they will take the taste, that's best."

Urging children to clean their plates, to finish every last morsel, can interfere with their developing ability to sense satiation, the feeling that makes a person end a meal. In a study comparing two groups of children, those who were taught to focus on noticing the sensation of fullness in their stomachs did better at adjusting their intake in response to foods' calorie density than the group rewarded for cleaning their plates. Children's bodies have their own well-regulated systems for determining their caloric needs. Those needs may vary from day to day—much to the distress of parents who want to see a child eat three "good" meals daily—but research has shown that even picky toddlers eat an appropriate and consistent number of calories for their size when their intake is averaged over two or three days. When a baby refuses to eat another spoonful or when a child says he is full, parents should respect the child's internal satiety signals. As soon as they are old enough to do so, children should be encouraged to determine their own portion sizes and serve themselves.

How else can parents and other adults best encourage healthy eating habits while avoiding battles over food? They can start by ensuring that the entire family is committed to having healthy foods in the home. The available choices, the menu at meals, and family policies about eating should be the same for everybody. Parents should not set a bad example by eating junk food or following an unbalanced fad diet while expecting their children to follow a different set of rules. Conversely, parents or other caregivers should not give in to the temptation to feed kids unhealthy items just because they are easy to prepare or because they know children will eat every bite. "It's essential" that the whole family commit to following a healthy eating plan, says Harvard's David Ludwig. "With overwhelming environmental influences to eat junk food and not get enough exercise, one has only the family. The family is the last bastion of defense against the toxic environment."

Children need to be able to control how much they eat and whether or not they will eat specific foods, but adults should determine what the range of choices in the pantry will be and what products will not be on the home menu. That strategy will help prevent battles over whether a child can or cannot have a particular food. It also encourages kids to develop healthy tastes that will persist as they get older. "Parents should be in charge of what children are offered and when, and children should be responsible for the decision to consume what is offered or not," write William Dietz of the CDC and Steven Gortmaker of the Harvard School of Public Health. "That division of responsibility is crucial," says Dietz. "Once the parents have made the offer, their responsibilities are over. If the child decides not to eat it, it's not the obligation of the parent to provide an alternative—which is always the temptation."

Parents whose child refuses to eat dinner may worry that the child will go to bed hungry. "I'd say, that's just the point," Dietz says. "Your child needs to learn the logical consequences of not eating. That's a lesson that many children never learn." Dietz believes that working parents who have limited time to spend with their kids may be tempted to give in to food demands because they think that having quality time with their children means avoiding an argument at any cost. "I think parents accede to their children's wishes about food when children are not in a position to make responsible decisions about food," he says, adding that, while there is no formal scientific evidence that the approach he advocates can reduce obesity, "it clearly reduces conflicts around feeding."

What kinds of foods can be considered "healthy" options? What kinds of products should parents and others who care for children choose to stock the refrigerator and pantry in order to promote good nutrition? Here too there's a good deal of agreement among nutrition experts. But before I offer specific suggestions, let's consider some basic information about the three major sources of energy that make up a balanced diet.

Energy-providing nutrients in food fall into three major categories: carbohydrates, proteins, and fats. Carbohydrates are sugars, present either as small molecules like glucose, fructose, and sucrose (table sugar)—the ingredients that sweeten baked goods, candy, and soft drinks—or linked together into much larger molecules called starches (as in potatoes, bread, rice, and pasta). Proteins are long, chainlike molecules found in animal products (meat, eggs, fish, dairy foods) but also in some plant foods such as tofu, brown rice, and beans. Fats are oily substances found both in animal products (meat, chicken, fish, butter, milk) and in many plant foods (avocadoes, nuts, olives, coconuts). Some foods belong strictly to one category—for instance, most fruits provide all or almost all of their calories from carbohydrates, while olive oil is pure fat. Many foods contain nutrients belonging to more than one category.

Our bodies are also partly made of proteins, fats, and, to a lesser degree, carbohydrates. For example, some 10,000 different kinds of proteins—molecules made of smaller building blocks called amino acids—provide the structural scaffolding for all of our cells and tissues as well as the chemical machinery (in the form of enzymes, hormones, neurotransmitters, and other substances) that keeps us alive and conscious of our environment. Fat is the major ingredient in the membranes that enclose and protect our cells, and it forms the insulation that sheathes nerves in the brain, spinal cord, and elsewhere in the body, allowing them to transmit messages rapidly. Sugars are attached to some of our bodies' important proteins and are sometimes found on the surfaces of our cells. For example, sugars are key components of the "blood group" proteins on the surfaces of red blood cells that determine whether a person's blood is type A, B, AB, or O. Fat and sugars are also stored in body tissues as energy depots.

Much of the seemingly inexhaustible debate about diets reported in the media centers on what proportion of daily calories people should get from each of the three major nutrient categories. Perhaps the most frequent topic of dispute concerns the percentage that should be obtained from fat. A related controversy centers on carbohydrates, the nutrient category that provides the majority of calories in most people's diets.

When the USDA's familiar Food Guide Pyramid, a teaching tool developed to illustrate the government's dietary guidelines, was first released in 1992, the average American got about 45 percent of daily calories from carbohydrates, about 40 percent from fat, and about 15 percent from protein. The dietary guidelines, at least since the early 1990s, have sought to reduce people's fat intake and to replace some of the fat calories with calories obtained from carbohydrates. Carbohydrates formed the base of the Food Guide Pyramid, with grain-based foods such as breads, cereals, and pastas recommended to provide at least half of one's daily calories. They also generally urged that fat intake be kept at no more than about 30 percent of daily calories. Protein made up the remaining 15 percent of daily caloric intake.

In the past decade or so, Americans have responded by reducing the proportion of calories they obtain from fat to about 35 percent, on average. They have also shifted their eating patterns to include many more reduced-fat and fat-free products. Such products are not always low calorie; often they simply provide their calories in the form of sugar or other carbohydrates instead of fat. During the same period, an increasing proportion of the population has become overweight or obese.

Some nutrition experts have speculated about whether the federal guidelines and their graphic representation in the Food Guide Pyramid might have unintentionally contributed to rising obesity rates by prompting people to eat too many carbohydrates, especially highly processed or refined carbohydrates that are quickly digested to sugar in the body. The food industry, in response to the government's recommendations, developed and marketed many new "low-fat" products that were high in such carbohydrates. The recent popularity of the Atkins and South Beach diets, weight-loss regimens that specify a relatively low percentage of calories from carbohydrates, has focused intense public attention on this nutrient category, making "low-carb" the latest marketing buzzword. Most dietitians would agree that cutting intake from some sources of carbohydrates—such as added sugars and highly processed starches, like those found in pastries, white bread, and pizza—would be healthy for many Americans. But carbohydrates from foods such as fruits, vegetables, whole grains, and beans should remain a healthy and fundamental part of a balanced diet.

The government's dietary guidelines, which establish the direction for all government nutrition programs, are revised every five years. As this book went to press, the expert committee charged with proposing changes for the upcoming 2005 dietary guidelines issued its recommendations. Regarding carbohydrates, the expert panel urges Americans to increase their fruit and vegetable intake and to opt for foods that are rich in fiber—for example, by choosing whole grains rather than refined grains and whole fruits rather than juices. It also notes the evidence linking sugar-sweetened beverages and weight gain, and suggests that reducing intake of added sugars (especially sugar-sweetened beverages) may help people control their weight.

🐜🐜🐜

How much fat should be included in a healthy diet? Some nutrition experts, such as Walter Willett of Harvard Medical School, argue in favor of allowing a somewhat higher fat intake than the current guidelines suggest—up to about 35 percent of daily calories instead of 30 percent—but emphasize that most of the fats people eat should come from plant oils and seafood rather than animal sources, as in the so-called Mediterranean diet (traditional in coastal areas of Italy, Greece, and Spain). Citing epidemiological and clinical studies, Willett contends that eating a moderate amount of these "healthy" fats helps prevent heart disease by raising HDL ("good") cholesterol. Willett and some of his colleagues have devised a food pyramid that reflects this advice.

The animal fat found in milk, butter, ice cream, cheese, and red meat is mostly of a type called saturated fat. Saturated fats are solid at room temperature; this property is related to the chemical structure of the carbon-chain molecules called fatty acids they are made of. In saturated fats, those carbon chains are maximally loaded with hydrogen atoms. A high intake of saturated fat raises the levels of total cholesterol, both LDL (nicknamed "bad" cholesterol because it can promote damage to arteries) and HDL (protective for arteries). On balance, a diet high in saturated fat increases the risk of chronic damage to the walls of arteries, a process that eventually causes narrowing of the blood vessels and leads to heart disease. Experts agree that Americans should limit their intake of saturated fats.

In contrast, unsaturated fats (both "monounsaturated" and "polyunsaturated") contain fatty acids composed of carbon chains that don't hold so many hydrogen atoms. These types of fats, which are liquid at room temperature, are the kind found in most vegetable oils, fish oil, and nuts. They are a healthier form of fat; in fact, research indicates that monounsaturated fats, especially, help protect against blood vessel damage. Both monounsaturated fats and polyunsaturated fats lower the blood level of "bad" LDL cholesterol and raise the level of "good" HDL cholesterol. There is widespread agreement that when possible the fats we eat should be monounsaturated or polyunsaturated. Especially healthy for the heart and blood vessels are the n-3 fatty acids, a class of polyunsaturated fatty acids found in fish, flaxseed and canola oils, walnuts, and various other foods. In any case, total fat intake should remain low to moderate.

A third fat category, trans fats, contains substances developed by the food industry as a way to artificially solidify fats from vegetable oil, making them more convenient to use in some kinds of cooking and prolonging the shelf life of certain products. Trans fats are made by chemically attaching some hydrogen atoms to the unsaturated carbon chains that make up vegetable fats. It turns out that trans fats are probably even worse for the arteries than saturated fats, because they raise LDL cholesterol but do not raise HDL cholesterol. Experts agree that people should try to avoid trans fats, which are present in stick margarine, in many fried foods, and in countless processed foods, such as commercial baked goods like crackers, bread, and cookies. It has been difficult for consumers to find out whether a product contained trans fats, but the Food and Drug Administration (FDA) has ruled that food companies must list them on product labels by 2006. Some companies have already begun to list the trans fat content on their labels or to identify products containing no trans fats. Mention of "partially hydrogenated vegetable oil" on a food label is another clue that a product contains trans fats.

Nutrition expert David Katz of the Prevention Research Center at Yale suggests that the debate among researchers over what level of fat intake is desirable has made people lose sight of a much more important point: most Americans can improve their diet by both reducing total fat intake and shifting away from saturated and trans fats. Epidemiological studies point to health benefits from both the Mediterranean diet and a traditional Asian diet, which is lower in fat. Trials of low-fat diets for prevention of heart attacks and diabetes have found that such diets are effective for those purposes. "We've got good evidence that cutting fat and shifting to healthy fats are both potentially good things to do," Katz says.

On the issue of dietary fat, the advisory panel for the government's 2005 dietary guidelines urges Americans to keep their daily saturated fat intake below 10 percent of total calories, to keep trans fat intake below 1 percent of total calories, and to eat no more than 300 milligrams of cholesterol per day. (Eggs and organ meats are rich in choles-

Types of Dietary Fat

	Main Sources	Effect on Cholesterol Compared with Carbohydrates
Monounsaturated	Olives and olive oil, canola oil, peanut oil; cashews, almonds, peanuts, and most other nuts; peanut butter; avocadoes	Lowers LDL; raises HDL
Polyunsaturated	Corn, soybean, safflower, and cottonseed oils; fish	Lowers LDL; raises HDL
Saturated	Whole milk, butter, cheese, and ice cream; red meat; chocolate; coconuts, coconut milk, and coconut oil	Raises both LDL and HDL
Trans	Most margarines; vegetable shortening; partially hydrogenated vegetable oil; deep-fried chips; many fast foods; most commercial baked goods	Raises LDL*

*Compared to monounsaturated or polyunsaturated fat, trans fat increases LDL, decreases HDL, and increases triglycerides.
Source: See Notes.

terol; it is also present in the fat found in meat, shellfish, poultry, and dairy products.) The panel also suggests eating 2 servings of fish a week because the n-3 fatty acids found in fish can help prevent heart disease, although it recommends that children and pregnant or breastfeeding women should avoid fish with a high mercury content. For adults the panel states that total fat intakes ranging from 20 percent to 35 percent are recommended—reflecting the idea expressed by Katz that both low-fat and moderate-fat diets can be acceptable, provided that the diet emphasizes "healthy" fats. However, very low fat diets are not recommended for children and adolescents. The panel recommends that children aged 2 to 3 years should get at least 30 percent of daily calories from fat and that children aged 4 to 18 should get at least 25 percent of calories from fat.

There is probably the least debate about protein, the third major source of nutrients in a balanced diet. A certain amount of daily protein in the diet is essential, since the human body cannot make all the amino acids it needs to stay alive and healthy. But the typical American diet contains ample protein for this purpose. Although the Atkins diet, a perennially popular short-term weight-loss diet, specifies a high percentage of calories from protein (as well as a low percentage from carbohydrates and a relatively high percentage from fat), many experts worry that eating a high-protein diet over a long period of time is potentially risky. It can cause calcium loss from the bones and places extra stress on the kidneys, which must excrete the waste compounds produced by digesting protein. (Following the Atkins diet for a long time is also likely to be hazardous for the heart and blood vessels, if people maintain a high total and saturated fat intake.)

All of this discussion about nutrient intake doesn't mean you have to sit down and figure out exactly what percentage of your daily calories comes from fat, carbohydrates, and protein. Such precision isn't necessary. An authoritative report on dietary intake was issued in 2002 by the Institute of Medicine. It reflects the current consensus among nutrition experts that various kinds of diets, including diets with a range of different intakes within the three major nutrient categories, can be healthy. Such a range reflects cultural variations in eating habits and recognizes that different individuals or families will prefer different foods. The report specifies that acceptable fat intakes can range from 20 percent to 35 percent of daily calories, carbohydrate intakes from 45 percent to 65 percent, and protein intakes from 10 percent to 35 percent. Anyone who sticks to the general eating principles about which there is broad agreement—emphasizing fruits and vegetables, whole grains and fiber, limiting foods with added sugars, and limiting total fat, especially unhealthy saturated or trans fats—should be able to eat a healthy diet.

Reducing or eliminating certain foods from the home still leaves ample room for variety. For example, parents can change their household shopping and cooking practices to limit red meats high in saturated fat, to include more fish, poultry, and vegetarian dishes, and to grill, bake, or steam foods instead of frying them. For snacks, children should be offered a choice, but everything on the list should be healthy: for example, fresh fruit, carrot sticks, dry-roasted nuts, whole wheat crackers with low-fat cheese, baked potato chips, raisins, low-fat yogurt, baked pretzels. Examples of items to be removed from kitchen shelves (and hence not available as a focus of conflict) might be fried chips, candy, and high-fat baked goods. If parents make a point of not buying calorie-dense sweets and snack foods loaded with unhealthy saturated or trans fats, children will not expect to eat them at home and will be more likely to develop a liking for healthier alternatives. Providing what David Katz calls "a safe nutritional environment" requires parents to become expert shoppers and label readers. "Know what to choose," he says. "If your kids want chips, you have chips. If they want cookies, you have cookies. But it's the best product in every category."

Many experts recommend that parents banish regular sodas and sugared drinks (such as fruit punch or fruit drinks containing a low percentage of fruit juice) from the household since they are a major source of "added sugars" in the diet unaccompanied by more valuable vitamins or nutrients. Although such drinks are high calorie, research suggests they do not trigger a corresponding sense of satiety, so drinking large quantities of them can greatly boost daily calorie intake.

Children, like adults, should be encouraged to drink water instead of sweetened beverages when they are thirsty. Many people tend to confuse thirst with hunger and reach for a soda when a glass of water is all they need. Keeping the body well hydrated is good for the kidneys, digestive tract, circulatory system, and brain, but drinking beverages that contain a lot of added sugar and minerals isn't really necessary, except perhaps for people who have been burning a great deal of energy or losing lots of sodium or potassium because of vigorous exercise or very hot weather. Teaching children to quench their thirst with water instead of with soft drinks and juices would go a long way toward reducing the calorie excess that is contributing to the obesity epidemic.

Milk is an important source of calcium for children, but kids older than 2 don't need whole milk. In fact, the only age group in America for whom whole milk is still considered healthy is children between 1 and 2 years old, because their brains are growing rapidly, and fat is the major ingredient in nerve cell membranes and the myelin that insulates nerves. On the other hand, infants under the age of 1 should receive breast milk or infant formula rather than cow's milk, because of concerns about links between early exposure to the proteins in cow's milk and allergies or other health problems.

Whole milk is almost 4 percent fat, which may not sound very high, but consider that about half the calories in whole milk come from fat, much of it the unhealthy saturated variety. For everyone over the age of 2, fat-free (skim) milk or milk that is 1 percent fat is a better choice. Similarly, choosing fat-free or low-fat yogurt, cheese, and cottage cheese will help limit saturated fat intake.

Two to three servings of dairy products per day for children and adults are recommended by current federal dietary guidelines. (Examples of a serving are a cup of milk or yogurt or an ounce and a half of low-fat cheese.) However, the advisory panel for the upcoming 2005 dietary guidelines recommends that adults and children should have approximately 3 cups daily of fat-free or low-fat milk or an equivalent amount of other nonfat or low-fat dairy products, particularly because of evidence that this level of dairy consumption can prevent low bone mass and osteoporosis in later life. Some epidemiological studies suggest that diets high in total calcium and dairy consumption may be associated with a reduced risk of obesity in children and adults. In a limited number of studies, dairy consumption has also been linked with a reduced risk of developing insulin resistance and the metabolic syndrome. Further research is needed to confirm these findings and to seek the explanations for them. For example, in some studies of children, higher dairy intake is associated with lower soda intake, a factor that might account for the observed reduction in obesity risk. On the other hand, laboratory studies in animals suggest that dietary calcium may play a role in fat cell metabolism, reducing the tendency to store fat and aiding in regulation of body weight. In addition, eating nonfat or low-fat dairy products may be associated with a reduced risk of obesity and of insulin resistance for other reasons besides calcium—for example, because such foods have a low glycemic index or because they may enhance satiety.

Some nutrition experts are skeptical of findings suggesting a link between dairy consumption and weight control, pointing out that much of the research has been funded by the dairy industry. A recent review of the evidence urges that large clinical trials be carried out in overweight adults to find out whether diets high in dairy products or total calcium can help people attain a healthier weight. Evidence from other epidemiological studies suggests that diets high in dairy products may be associated with a small increase in the risk in later life of prostate cancer (a common cancer in older men) and ovarian cancer (a rare one in women). Since studies exploring these possible associations have yielded inconsistent results, further research is needed to determine whether they are meaningful. On balance, milk and other dairy foods provide valuable nutrients and help build and maintain bone strength. It makes sense for children and adults to include them in their diet as long they are careful to choose fat-free or low-fat products.

Not everyone can digest dairy products easily. Babies, of course, are engineered to digest everything in breast milk, and most young children can digest cow's milk, although some are allergic to certain proteins in it. However, many teens and adults have trouble digesting dairy foods because their bodies make reduced quantities of the enzyme lactase, which breaks down lactose, the major sugar in milk. People with reduced lactase levels can suffer nausea, cramps, bloating, gas, or diarrhea after drinking milk or eating other dairy products; but there are some who find that they can eat a few select dairy foods and others who never develop any symptoms. Population studies indicate that lactose intolerance, as this condition is called, is present in as many as 75 percent of African Americans and American Indians, and 90 percent of Asian Americans. People with lactose intolerance can take lactase tablets or drops when they eat dairy foods to aid digestion, and reduced-lactose dairy products are also available.

In addition to dairy products, other good sources of dietary calcium include canned sardines and salmon, calcium-fortified soy milk, calcium-fortified orange juice, and broccoli.

An area of striking unanimity among nutrition experts is the paramount importance of daily fruits and vegetables. They provide calories (mostly in the form of carbohydrates) along with abundant vitamins, fiber, and natural anticancer substances. A wealth of epidemiological evidence has linked high vegetable and fruit intake with a reduced risk of heart disease, stroke, diabetes, and various kinds of cancer, including cancers of the mouth and throat, lung, stomach, bladder, colon, breast, and prostate. People who regularly eat lots of fruits and vegetables have a lower frequency of constipation and gastrointestinal disorders and even gain some protection against cataracts and macular degeneration, two eye disorders common in old age.

Walter Willett of Harvard suggests in his book *Eat, Drink and Be Healthy* that the USDA's "5 A Day" campaign, aimed at increasing Americans' intake of fruits and vegetables, has somewhat misled the public by setting the bar too low. Five servings a day is the minimum recommended by national dietary guidelines, which set the serving number as a proportion of total daily calories. Children over 6, teenage girls, active women, and most men are supposed to get 7 servings a day, while teenage boys and physically active men are supposed to eat 9. For the forthcoming 2005 dietary guidelines, an advisory panel has recommended further boosting recommended daily vegetable and fruit intake. The panel advises that Americans should consume between 5 and 13 servings daily, with the recommended number for different age groups dependent on overall calorie needs.

Willett also believes that potatoes (America's most popular "vegetable") should not even be counted in figuring one's daily vegetable servings because they are mostly starch and ought to belong to the bread and grain category. He suggests striving for color and variety in the diet by including offerings from several categories (dark green leafy vegetables, yellow or orange fruits and vegetables, red fruits and vegetables, beans, and citrus fruits). Fresh produce should be washed under cold running tap water before it is eaten or cooked to remove dirt, bacteria, and other residues. Vegetables with a hard surface, such as potatoes or carrots, can be scrubbed with a brush. In a large, federally funded randomized trial, Dietary Approaches to Stop Hypertension, or DASH, researchers found that a diet containing 8 to 10 servings of fruits and vegetables per day was very effective in reducing blood pressure among people whose pressure was high enough to need medical treatment. In addition, most vegetables and fruits contain healthful fiber and have a low glycemic index: they tend to fill people up without causing rapid surges in blood sugar or insulin levels. The more of them we eat, the healthier we as a population are likely to be.

Experts, including the advisory panel for the 2005 dietary guidelines, also concur that Americans should boost their intake of whole grains and fiber. One of the best sources of fiber, whole grains also contain vitamins, minerals, and healthy unsaturated fats. Many of these valuable components are lost when grains are cracked and milled to remove their outer layers and the plant embryo portion of the seed, such as during the manufacture of white flour from whole wheat. Eating whole grains reduces the risk of diabetes, heart disease, and several kinds of cancer and prevents constipation. By switching to brown rice or whole grain pasta and by choosing breads, crackers, and cereals that list "whole wheat," "whole oats," "whole rye," or another whole grain as the first ingredient on the label, families can easily incorporate more whole grains in their diets.

Fiber—also abundant in fresh fruits and vegetables and dried beans or legumes—is healthy for many reasons. It helps prevent overeating by contributing to a sense of fullness at mealtime. It keeps blood sugar from rising too fast by slowing down digestion and absorption of sugars. A high-fiber diet reduces the risk of diabetes and heart disease and prevents constipation. Some fiber remains solid (insoluble) in the digestive tract, helping make stools softer and bulkier; other fiber dissolves in intestinal fluid and traps bile acids that contain cholesterol, thereby lowering the blood level of cholesterol.

So far I have been describing *what* to eat as part of a healthy diet. Traditionally, that has also been the focus of the nutrition lessons children get in school. But many dietitians and educators now believe that an important piece has been left out: teaching people *how much* to eat—and how to avoid overeating.

Research suggests that without realizing it Americans have shifted to consuming larger portions than they need, perhaps as a result of the "supersizing" phenomenon mentioned earlier. Parents and others who feed children can do a lot to reverse this unhealthy trend by teaching kids (and in the process themselves) how to estimate appropriate portions. The easiest starting point is to learn about standard serving sizes by reading the nutritional information on food packages or from other sources, such as the USDA Web site. The site has a helpful chart of serving sizes, along with other useful information such as the number of daily servings recommended for children of different ages. (See page 267 in Resources.) You may be surprised to discover that a "serving" of many foods is a lot smaller than you thought: for instance, 2 to 3 ounces of cooked meat or fish, 2 tablespoons of peanut butter, or 1 egg counts as a serving in the meat and beans (protein-containing) food group.

Try measuring family portion sizes at home for a few days to learn how to estimate serving sizes accurately. Figuring out how much food your cereal bowls and serving spoons actually hold will make you better at estimating. Children can help with this process and can learn how to determine the serving size by checking the nutrition labels of food packages. You can also use handy tricks. An adult's fist or a tennis ball is about the volume of 1 cup (which is 2 servings of pasta or rice). An adult's thumb from tip to base is about the size of 1 ounce of meat or cheese. An adult's palm minus the fingers, or a standard-sized audiocassette, is about the size of a 3-ounce serving of cooked meat, fish, or poultry. A handful of potato chips, pretzels, or raisins is about the size of 1 serving of those foods.

Nutrition scientist Barbara Rolls has done extensive research exploring how meal composition and environmental cues unconsciously affect people's capacity to regulate their food intake. Rolls's findings suggest that satiation tends to occur predictably when the individual has consumed a certain weight or volume of food, not a certain number of calories. For this reason, overconsumption is much more likely when people eat foods that are high-fat and therefore "calorie dense"—that is, containing more calories per unit of weight—than when they eat foods that are not calorie dense. Fat contains 9 calories per gram; protein and carbohydrate, 4 per gram; fiber, 1.5 to 2.5 calories per gram. Fresh vegetables and most fresh fruits have low calorie density because much of their weight is water (no calories) and fiber. Water-based soups also have a low calorie density.

Rolls's findings form the basis for a practical, relatively low-fat approach to eating that anyone can adopt to avoid overconsuming calories. As she explains in her book *Volumetrics,* a key strategy is to make meals and snacks less energy dense by including lots of fresh vegetables, fruits, and fiber and by incorporating water into food (for instance, in soups, stews, and cooked grains). Much current sound nutrition advice is based on similar principles. For example, some experts recommend dividing each person's dinner plate into imaginary sections, with two-thirds of the space devoted to vegetables, whole grains, and/or beans and one-third or less assigned to the animal protein portion. Others suggest serving salad, soup, or vegetables first (when the family is hungriest) and grain and/or protein portions afterward. Low-fat salads (made without too much dressing) help fill people up and keep them from overconsuming the more calorie dense foods on the menu. Serving vegetables and any unfamiliar or "new" foods first also makes it more likely that children will eat some of those items.

David Katz suggests using the "stoplight" concept popularized by pediatric obesity treatment expert Leonard Epstein as a tool to teach everybody better eating habits. He feels it could even be used on food labels. In this scheme, foods in the "green" category, such as vegetables, fruits, and some whole grains that are low in energy density and high in nutrients, can be eaten in large quantities. Most foods are "yellow," with moderate energy density and nutrient content; they should be eaten regularly in moderation. "Red" foods, such as desserts, are high in calories and low in nutrients and should be eaten as treats, in small quantities. It's a good idea to keep plenty of "green" foods visible in the kitchen and refrigerator for kids to grab when they're looking for a snack.

At David Ludwig's OWL clinic in Boston, the eating plan that was taught to Adam and his family uses a somewhat different approach based on foods' glycemic index—but there too the goal is to help children achieve and maintain a healthy weight by avoiding overconsumption of calories. Like Rolls's volumetrics strategy, it's meant to be a long-term approach to eating, not a temporary measure. The concept of foods' glycemic index originated as a way of studying how various foods affected the ups and downs of blood sugar in people with diabetes. Researchers reasoned that since some foods raise blood glucose levels faster and higher than others, designing a diabetic person's diet to include foods with a low glycemic index might be useful as part of treatment. Such a diet might cause smaller swings in blood glucose levels and thereby allow diabetics to reduce the dose of injected insulin. One of the earliest studies on the concept, published in 1983 in the *New England Journal of Medicine,* contained the surprising finding that eating a potato raised blood glucose levels as rapidly as eating a comparable amount of carbohydrate in the form of sugar. Since the 1980s about a dozen studies have indeed found that low-glycemic-index diets improve blood sugar control in diabetes. Although such diets are not yet routinely recommended by the American Diabetes Association, which cites the need for additional research, the approach has been endorsed by diabetes associations in several other countries.

Even in nondiabetics, there is reason to suspect that the big boost in blood glucose caused by meals full of high-glycemic-index carbohydrates may not be healthy. Such foods (potatoes, white bread, sweets, bagels, and many other baked goods, for example) send blood glucose level rapidly upward, triggering abundant release of insulin. Insulin's message to the body is, store these calories immediately! In response, glucose is quickly taken up by muscle cells and by the liver (which conserves it as a starch called glycogen), while free fatty acids in the bloodstream are quickly sopped up by fat cells. Within a few hours the body's efficient storage action makes blood glucose drop steeply. Since the brain needs a constant supply of glucose to function, the sudden drop sets off alarm signals, instructing the system to switch gears from storing energy to making it available. Another set of hormones—epinephrine, glucagons, cortisol, and growth hormone—brings the blood's glucose level back up to within a more normal level. Ludwig's research suggests that one of the actions of these hormones is to trigger intense hunger for the next meal.

In one study Ludwig and several colleagues divided 12 obese teenage boys into three groups and fed each group a different test meal. Two of the meals were identical in total calories and in the proportion of calories that came from each category of nutrient, but one had a medium glycemic index (for instance, it contained steel-cut oatmeal) and one had a high glycemic index (it contained instant oatmeal). The third test meal had exactly the same number of calories as the other two but contained foods with a low glycemic index: a vegetable omelet and fresh fruit. Everyone in a group received that group's test meal for both breakfast and lunch. The participants' levels of glucose, fatty acids, insulin, and other hormones were measured at intervals after the meals. The boys were asked to rate their hunger level at various times throughout the day. During the five-hour period after lunch, food was freely available and the participants' requests for food and food intake were recorded.

The high-glycemic-index meal provoked a much bigger and more sustained rise in glucose than the low-glycemic-index meal and a correspondingly greater surge in insulin. By five hours after breakfast the blood glucose levels of boys who had eaten the high-glycemic-index meal had plummeted to below their original fasting levels, while the glucose levels in boys who ate the low-glycemic-index meal had come down only gradually, reaching about the original fasting level. Throughout the day, boys who ate the high-glycemic-index meal reported greater hunger than those in the other two groups. By the end of the day (after snacking in the afternoon on food that was freely available to all groups), the boys given the high-glycemic-index meal had eaten 81 percent more total calories than the boys given the low-glycemic-index meal. Those given the medium-glycemic-index meal had eaten 53 percent more calories than the low-glycemic-index group. The implication of these findings is that eating lots of carbohydrates with a high glycemic index may put the body on a metabolic and hormonal seesaw whose net result is increased hunger and higher total calorie consumption. A calorie is still a calorie—and eating excess calories will cause weight gain, regardless of whether those calories come from carbohydrates, proteins, or fats, but the overall makeup of the diet might indirectly influence how many calories are ingested.

When the government began urging Americans to reduce their total fat intake, Ludwig notes, "the food industry came in and encouraged us to be eating low-fat foods that were high in starch and sugar, instead of [promoting] fruits and vegetables. You can't brand broccoli as easily as you can muffins. When fat got replaced by starch and sugar rather than by fruits and vegetables, the bargain may have been a bad one for body weight regulation."

Ludwig's research on how the body adapts to a calorie-restricted diet aimed at producing weight loss suggests that a low-glycemic-index diet might be less likely than a high-glycemic-index diet to trigger counterproductive physiological defenses against weight loss. For instance, in a recent 12-month study, 16 overweight teenagers were randomly assigned either to a calorie-restricted low-fat diet (25 to 30 percent fat, 55 to 60 percent carbohydrate) or to a low-to-moderate-glycemic-index diet (30 to 35 percent fat, 45 to 50 percent carbohydrate). Those in the low-glycemic-index group were counseled to include some protein and fat along with their carbohydrates at every meal and snack, but unlike the low-fat group, their calories were not restricted: they were told to eat until they were satisfied and to snack when hungry. Both groups received identical behavioral therapy and physical activity recommendations, and both followed their diets for six months. Then they were monitored for another six months. Seven participants in each group completed the study. At the end of one year, those in the low-glycemic-index group (despite the lack of calorie restriction) had lost significantly more weight and more fat—11 pounds more on average—than those in the low-fat group.

In the competition among nutrition researchers over how to build a better food pyramid, David Ludwig and his colleague Cara B. Ebbeling have their own entry. It reflects a diet based on foods with a low glycemic load (a term that reflects both a food's glycemic index and its total carbohydrate content). Unlike the USDA Food Guide Pyramid, it makes fruits and vegetables the foundation. Grain-based foods have been moved farther up the pyramid and thus make up a smaller proportion of the diet than in the USDA version. Protein (in the form of nuts, dairy, poultry, and fish) is featured a bit more prominently.

No large long-term studies of low-glycemic-index diets have yet been conducted. Some experts are wary of advising consumers to use the glycemic index as a tool for choosing what to eat. They note that any food's impact on the blood glucose level depends not only on its glycemic index but on the quantity consumed and on whether it is eaten along with other foods that might slow the absorption of nutrients from the intestinal tract. Nutrition researcher William Dietz says he is not convinced that foods' low glycemic index accounts for the weight loss seen among participants in Ludwig's studies. "I think the diets induce weight loss, but I question whether it's the glycemic index or the high water content of the fruits and vegetables in the diet," Dietz says.

Parents and other consumers can leave the wrangling over details to the nutrition scientists. There is practical wisdom to be extracted from the research of Rolls, Ludwig, Willett, and others—and their take-home messages are not really so far apart. Boiled down to essentials, the kinds of foods recommended for a low-glycemic-index diet are not especially radical; in fact, they fit easily within the framework of the general noncontroversial dietary advice detailed earlier in this chapter. As Ludwig summarized his basic instructions in a recent medical article, "Increase consumption of fruits, vegetables and legumes (beans), choose grain products processed according to traditional rather than modern methods (pasta, stone-ground breads, old-fashioned oatmeal, for example), and limit intake of potatoes and concentrated sugar."

There's plenty of common ground among nutrition experts, and consumers can't go wrong by basing their diet on the areas of consensus. Eat lots of fresh vegetables and fruits, whole grains, and fiber. Choose fat-free or low-fat dairy products. Maintain a moderate protein intake. Substitute "healthy" fats for unhealthy ones. Limit total fat intake. Cut back on foods and drinks that are high in added sugars, fat, or highly processed carbohydrates. These are the lessons the science teaches. It's not so hard for a family to apply them and adopt a healthy way of eating. As Adam says, "It's one of the easiest things I do."

CHAPTER 5

Off the Couch and Away from the Screen

I t's time for Nancy Driscoll's second-grade class to study language arts. Like second-graders in many U.S. schools, they are learning about synonyms and antonyms: words with similar meanings and with opposite meanings. But unlike kids in most other elementary schools, these students are not about to take their lesson sitting down. "Stand by your desks," Driscoll orders the children. "If I say two words and they're synonyms, jump and clap five times. If I say two words that are antonyms, do five lunges." And if the words are homonyms—sounding the same but with different meanings—the students are instructed to touch their toes five times.

The children stand by their desks as the lesson begins. While the teacher calls out each pair of words, the kids rhythmically punch the air five times. Next, they snap their fingers five times in unison to mark their "think time" before jumping, lunging, or touching toes.

"Friend, enemy," Driscoll calls out. Punch. Snap. Lunge.

"Sick, ill." Punch. Snap. Everybody jumps and claps.

"Dear, deer." Punch. Snap. Up and down the students bob, fingers stretching to toes.

The words keep coming and the kids keep moving, literally thinking on their feet as they figure out how to respond to each pair. The task requires concentration, and there's no talking or laughing, just the steady beat of 15 second-graders jumping, clapping, or bouncing up and down.

After several minutes of this drill, Driscoll rewards them by picking each child in turn to choose and lead an exercise. Now the kids giggle as they follow the leader, twisting, pretending to jump rope, or briefly dropping to the floor to do push-ups. When they've been moving around for a total of 10 minutes, it's back to their seats. Smiling and energized now, they're ready for whatever Driscoll does next.

These students at Brookridge Elementary, part of the Shawnee Mission School District in suburban Kansas City, Kansas, are participating in an innovative three-year experiment, involving several thousand Kansas elementary school children, aimed at finding out whether building physical activity into academic lessons during the school day can help prevent children from becoming overweight. The Kansas project reflects a growing consensus among researchers and health experts that in order to turn back the childhood obesity epidemic, Americans will have to do more than just make sure their kids are taking a gym class. They will also have to find creative new ways to build more physical activity into their children's daily routines—and into their own.

Efforts to reduce obesity levels by ramping up school physical education programs have so far failed. Even when students are given intensified P.E. classes, most studies have found that they do not get enough minutes per week of exercise during P.E. to make an impact. And around the nation, physical education time and even recess breaks are increasingly casualties of the pervasive pressure on schools to pack more academic lessons and test preparation into students' days. Yet educators are beginning to acknowledge that schools must do their part in fighting the growing problem of childhood obesity.

That's why University of Kansas researchers, with federal funding from the National Institutes of Health, embarked in the fall of 2003 on a program called Physical Activity Across the Curriculum, or PAAC. Their hope is that PAAC will accomplish dual goals: prove it's possible for classroom teachers to get kids moving and to help protect them from becoming overweight, and show that children's activity levels can be increased during the school day without cutting into academic time. Unlike some previous programs, PAAC is specifically designed not to require teachers to schedule "exercise breaks" that are separate from instruction. "If it's three minutes here and three minutes there, that's fine," says Janet May, PAAC project coordinator for Kansas City schools during the program's first year. "We want them to incorporate it into learning."

Researchers caution that it is still too soon to say whether such an approach can succeed, but if PAAC is effective, its concepts could ultimately influence the methods of teachers nationwide. In time PAAC and other programs like it could lead to a shift in classroom routines that makes learning a more physically active process. "The key concept here is that there is no loss of academic instruction time," explains Joseph E. Donnelly, a professor of exercise science at the University of Kansas who is leading the project. "You take your existing lesson and instead of talking your way through it, you move your way through it."

Teachers at the PAAC schools in the Kansas City area and in Topeka receive training and support, including myriad suggestions in a manual and on a Web site, for including physical activity in lessons about any subject—math, social studies, language arts, science. Janet May says much of the training is designed to help teachers realize how easy it is to do so, especially for students in the early elementary grades. "The best ideas come right from the teacher," she notes.

At Briarwood Elementary, another PAAC school in the Shawnee Mission district, Susan Reichardt's third-grade class has been studying the human body. "I want you to get up, push in your chair, and make your blood pump faster," says Reichardt. Some students start doing jumping jacks, others jump up and down or run in place.

"Now move a hinge joint," she orders. They flex their elbows.

"Move a ball joint." They swing their arms around.

"Now do a pivot on a pivot joint." They swivel their hips, pretending to swing a bat.

Incorporating activity becomes a greater challenge in the upper elementary grades, when students must master more complex subject matter, but teachers participating in PAAC are finding ways to do it. In another Briarwood classroom, Marsha Plese is teaching her fifth-graders how to form the possessive of plural nouns. She calls a student named Anna to the front of the class to demonstrate what she wants. To act out an apostrophe, Anna does a side stretch. To make an "s," she does a deep knee bend. Plese explains to her class that plural nouns ending in "s," like "doctors," need only an apostrophe to make the possessive form: "doctors'." But some other plural nouns, like "men," require both an apostrophe and an "s": "men's." As she calls out various words, her students act out the answers.

Teachers in the PAAC program are asked to include 100 minutes of physical activity each week in their academic lessons, deciding for themselves how to apportion the minutes. The project has enrolled 24 Kansas elementary schools, of which 14 are "intervention" schools (incorporating physical activity into lessons) and 10 are "control" schools (following their usual educational programs and serving as a comparison). Donnelly observes that school principals were not drawn to the program because of its potential health benefits. Researchers found that the most effective way to promote PAAC to school officials was by providing evidence that physical activity could improve academic performance, appeal to diverse learning styles, and make children calmer and more manageable. "We got nowhere when our rap was all about diabetes and obesity," Donnelly recalls. "Everybody said, 'That's important, but what does it have to do with us?'"

In all of the schools, second- and third-graders were weighed and measured at the start of the program, and their BMIs were recorded. A subset of students in these grades have also undergone more detailed testing, including blood tests to measure levels of glucose, insulin, cholesterol, and other components, blood pressure testing, measurement of waist and hip circumference, measurement of skin-fold thicknesses to estimate fat stores, cognitive testing by psychologists, and a submaximal fitness test in which their heart rates are measured after they ride an exercise bicycle.

Throughout the program's three-year life, observers will randomly visit classrooms in intervention and control schools to assess students' physical activity levels during the day. At the end of the study, all students will again have their BMIs measured to determine whether incorporating regular physical activity into lessons reduced obesity rates in the intervention schools. In addition, researchers will find out whether PAAC has an impact on students' overall physical fitness, cognitive ability, blood pressure, cholesterol, or other health factors.

In a mobile clinic parked behind Prairie Elementary School, members of the PAAC research team are doing fitness tests on third-grade students. Assistant Greg McMillan buckles a heart-rate monitor around the chest of Jacob, a serious-looking boy whose T-shirt reads "Take me to your candy." Greg asks him to start pedaling the exercise bike at a steady rate of 60 revolutions per minute. "We'll do this for a couple of minutes to let your muscles warm up. Then I'm going to change the gear like you're going up a steep hill."

Jacob's heart rate reaches 122 beats per minute, a healthy response to moderate exercise in a child his age, while he pedals the bike "on the flat." Greg then adjusts the bike to increase resistance. "He's fairly fit, so he gets a higher wattage," he explains. "Keep those legs pumping, Jacob. You've got to get up this hill. Come on, Jacob, you can do it. You're getting close to the top now." When Jacob's heart rate hits 171 beats per minute, the monitor beeps, signaling the end of the test. Greg dials down the resistance. Breathing hard, Jacob pedals slowly to cool down.

Donnelly and his team are uncertain whether the amount of classroom activity provided in PAAC will be sufficient to make children more physically fit, but they hope it will boost daily calorie expenditure enough to effect a measurable impact on obesity levels. Equally important, they hope that the program will produce a lasting change in students' attitudes about activity that might, over time, change norms in the U.S. population as a whole. After participating in PAAC, "we hope that when somebody is 30, they will think that they can be physically active any time, any place," Donnelly says.

🐜🐜🐜

America's children urgently need to get moving. Current national recommendations issued by the Institute of Medicine and by the National

Association for Sports and Physical Education call for children to accumulate a minimum of 60 minutes of moderate to vigorous physical activity each day. Yet surveys suggest that most children and teenagers in the United States don't come close to that level of activity. The lifestyle of most U.S. children today is far more sedentary than that of kids who grew up a few decades ago. The reasons are many and include sprawling suburbs that force dependence on cars; traffic and neighborhood conditions that make it difficult, dangerous, or impossible for many children to walk to school or to play outside; cutbacks in school physical education programs; work schedules that prevent many parents from being available to supervise after-school play; the lure of the passive entertainment provided by television, computers, and video games; the demands of homework and academic schedules; and the inadequacy of after-school sports and recreation programs.

Experts are unsure how much each of these factors contributes to children's inactivity and to rising obesity rates. They concur, however, that finding ways to make kids more physically active should be a central part of the strategy for turning back the obesity epidemic. Human bodies store fat whenever the calories they take in exceed the calories they burn. To restore balance to that equation and to prevent weight gain, a child (or an adult) must either eat fewer calories, expend more energy in physical activity, or both.

But what is physical activity? Most people would probably say it's exercise: playing a sport, working out, taking a physical education class. The true definition is far broader, encompassing everything children or adults do with their muscles from the moment they wake up in the morning until they go to sleep at night. It includes walking or biking to school, playing outside, walking the dog, doing household chores, playing on an after-school sports team, going swimming, climbing stairs, carrying a book-filled backpack, dancing around the living room, even fidgeting in class—as well as participating in sports or P.E. All of these activities burn calories and contribute to the dynamic balance between food intake and energy use that determines body weight.

Many experimental programs aimed at preventing or reducing obesity in children have focused on improving just one component of physical activity by offering longer and more vigorous P.E. classes at school or after-school sessions of group exercise or dance. So far, testing indicates that making a sizeable populationwide difference in children's activity levels—a difference substantial enough to help slow or stop the epidemic—will require changing more than just one component of what kids do. A concerted effort will probably be needed to offer children all kinds of opportunities and incentives to become more active, both in school and at home. Some research findings suggest that a key initial goal for many families might be reducing the time kids (and adults) spend watching TV, sitting at the computer, and playing video games each week and substituting other, more active ways to have fun.

Parents, teachers, child-care providers, youth group leaders, coaches, and others responsible for the welfare of children should be encouraged to think creatively about what children do during the day and about how those patterns can be tweaked to incorporate more movement. Kids can be part of that process, brainstorming to come up with ideas and incentives. At home the answers might include getting rid of a television set or putting kids on a TV allowance, signing up for a community soccer program, buying a push lawn mower, taking a dance class, giving children a larger share of household chores, leaving the family car in the garage on some mornings. Schools are increasingly being expected to participate in this effort. Some state governments have recently passed new laws requiring an increase in the number of minutes students spend weekly being physically active at school. Texas, for example, recently legislated 135 minutes of activity a week, a statewide policy change that has forced some classroom teachers to schedule and lead daily workouts.

Just as encouraging kids to develop healthy eating habits is a familywide endeavor, getting them to become more active also involves changing everyone's behavior patterns. Steven Gortmaker of Harvard has been tracking the pediatric obesity epidemic since the 1980s, as well as designing innovative school- and community-based strategies to combat it. He believes that Americans' current unhealthy eating habits and sedentary lifestyles have been promoted by powerful economic forces, including the food industry, advertising, the television and motion picture industries, and the makers of computers and video games.

Nevertheless he remains refreshingly optimistic about the chances of improving the outlook, especially for children. "The epidemic is driven by [the equivalent of] less than a can of soda a day," he says. "It's so rooted in everyday behaviors that when you take them one at a time, there's nothing wrong with them." Added together, however, those behaviors are making more and more children and adults overweight each year.

Getting kids to move more should be the easiest part of the solution, Gortmaker predicts. "The physical activity is the part of this that I think is going to be solved a lot quicker. Kids really enjoy playing and running around.... All we need to do is return to where we were about 25 years ago."

🐜🐜🐜

Precise information doesn't exist to quantify how active children are today compared with children a quarter-century ago. Recently researchers have begun using devices such as accelerometers and pedometers—electronic devices that can be worn on the body—to measure kids' activity levels. But until the past decade or so, almost all information on exercise and physical activity was self-reported, by people answering questionnaires—and most of it was collected on adults, not children.

National surveys of U.S. adults suggest that in spite of being urged in recent years to get more exercise, most Americans have not boosted their activity levels much during the past two decades. Between 1986 and 1997, the proportion of U.S. adults who reported no leisure-time physical activity (essentially synonymous, in those surveys, with exercise) stayed roughly constant at around one-third. A more recent national survey, conducted in 2000, was worded differently from previous ones but found no significant change in the percentage of adults who said they were physically active in their leisure time. It reported that men were more likely to be physically active than women and that whites more often engaged in high levels of physical activity than African Americans or Hispanics. People with incomes below the poverty level were three times more likely to be inactive than those in the highest income group. The most highly educated Americans were the group most likely to engage in regular vigorous activity.

In 2001 government researchers tried for the first time to measure how much physical activity Americans did as they went through their daily lives and added those figures to the activity totals that people reported from deliberate exercise. Preliminary results show that even with the addition of routine daily activities like stair climbing or walking around, more than half of American adults get less than 30 minutes of moderate exercise per day. ("Moderate" means enough to raise the heart rate and cause a little sweating, such as brisk walking.) About one-quarter of participants said they did no moderate physical activity.

If so many U.S. adults are couch potatoes, we shouldn't be surprised that our children appear to follow a similar pattern. Data comparing the daily activity levels of American kids with those of children in other countries were recently collected by Brigham Young University researchers, who distributed pedometers to a sample of about 2,000 schoolchildren in the United States, Sweden, and Australia. The kids, between 6 and 12 years old, wore the pedometers for four consecutive days so that the instruments could record their daily step totals. Youngsters were also weighed and measured. Researchers then calculated the average number of steps taken daily by participating children in each country.

Boys and girls from the United States were significantly less active and significantly heavier than those from the other two countries. The U.S. sample also showed a steeper increase in BMI with age than was seen in kids from Sweden or Australia. For example, average step counts for U.S. boys in the study ranged from 12,554 to 13,872, compared with average counts of 15,673 to 18,346 for the Swedish boys, the most active group. (The totals for Australian boys were intermediate.) One-third of the American boys in the study were classified as overweight, compared to about 16 percent of Swedish and Australian boys. The step counts for girls were lower than for boys, but the cross-country comparisons among girls revealed a similar pattern.

Judging by these step counts, American elementary school kids are considerably more active than American grownups: a recent survey found that U.S. adults average about 5,310 steps per day. Yet many children undoubtedly fail to meet even minimal recommendations on physical activity. A 1996 report of the U.S. Surgeon General recommends that all Americans over the age of 2 should get "at least 30 minutes of endurance-type physical activity, of at least moderate intensity, on most preferably all days of the week." Other expert bodies have concluded that 30 minutes is not enough, especially for kids. The National Association of Sport and Physical Education recommends that elementary school–age children spend at least 60 minutes a day doing moderate to vigorous physical activity. The Institute of Medicine recommends at least an hour of moderately intense activity daily for both children and adults.

Unlike kids a few decades ago, children in the United States today rarely walk or ride their bikes to school or to other destinations. Half are driven to school in cars and about one-third take buses. Less than one trip in seven is made on foot or by bicycle. In a recent survey long distances were most often cited as the reason why children went to school by car or bus, but traffic was a close second. Concerns about traffic danger prevent an estimated 20 million children in the United States from walking or biking to school.

Kids get between 20 percent and 40 percent of their total physical activity at school. School gym classes and recess periods provide the only strenuous exercise many U.S. children get during the week, yet studies suggest that at most schools the minutes children actually spend in vigorous activity are few indeed. Most children in grades 1 through 6 are enrolled in physical education, averaging about three class periods a week. But trained observers watching such classes as part of one research study found that students engaged in only about three minutes of moderate to vigorous exercise per class—less than 10 percent of total class time! Some experts have estimated that during the elementary grades children may average as little as 10 minutes per week of moderate to vigorous activity in school P.E. classes. Furthermore, most children are not taught by P.E. specialist teachers, and many school systems, strapped for funds, have severely cut their physical education budgets in recent years. In the Los Angeles Unified School District, California's largest, some P.E. classes in middle schools have more than 70 students per teacher. National guidelines recommend no more than 25 students per P.E. teacher. Fields and courts are so crowded that students spend much of their class time waiting their turn to run wind sprints or shoot baskets.

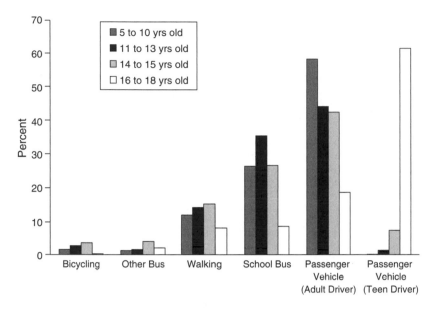

The percentage of trips during normal school travel hours. The majority of children arrive and leave school in automobiles, vans, trucks, and buses.
Source: See Notes.

When children are young, boys and girls are equally physically active, but as they move from childhood into adolescence, starting at about the age of 10, physical activity levels for both sexes—and especially for girls—begin to decline. Decreased emphasis on P.E. classes after elementary school probably contributes to part of the reduction. About half of U.S. schools require physical education for students in grades 1 through 5, but this percentage drops off steeply in the higher grades. Fewer than 10 percent of high schools require physical education for students in grades 10 through 12, even though P.E. programs have been shown to have a strong impact on activity levels in this age group. Higher family incomes, higher levels of maternal education, and access to a community recreation center are also linked to higher physical activity levels among adolescents, while those living in high-crime neighborhoods are less likely to be active.

Along with declining overall activity levels, adolescents of both sexes participate in fewer physically active leisure-time activities (such as basketball, bicycling, softball, running, and aerobics) as they get older. Why so many teenagers stop participating is not known, but the reasons could be related to academic pressure, exclusion from competitive sports programs, transportation problems, lack of parental support, a need to earn money after school, or the lure of sedentary forms of entertainment such as television and computer games. James F. Sallis, a professor of psychology at San Diego State University, suggests that high school sports programs, with their emphasis on competition and athletic prowess, take money away from physical education programs and paradoxically discourage many teenagers from remaining active and physically fit. High schools often require only one or two years of P.E., and the demands of academic schedules and extracurricular activities often make it difficult or impossible for kids to take more. "There's this pyramid, especially as kids get older," Sallis says. "If they're not the [athletic] elite, they are invited out. They are excluded. We think that this policy to pursue competition and winning, instead of promoting health in these kids, is actually contributing to the decline in activity with age. . . . The opportunities that are available to kids as they get older are diminished by design."

Yet daily physical education classes for all students are recommended by federal health guidelines and by the American Academy of Pediatrics (AAP). Daily P.E. classes, lasting 30 to 60 minutes, are recommended in the Institute of Medicine's 2005 report on preventing childhood obesity, which also urges schools to expand the array of physical activity choices, intramural sports, and clubs they offer, both during and after the regular school day, to meet the needs and interests of more students. The purpose of P.E., especially as children become adolescents, is not only to allow kids to exercise, but to give them the skills they need to play individual sports and develop personal fitness programs that they can continue to follow as adults. "It's quite rare that that's a focus in high school," remarks Sallis.

For girls in particular, the remarkable drop in physical activity that often accompanies adolescence may also be caused in part by biological factors that affect both energy expenditure and behavior. Between the ages of 10 and 18, activity levels fall by 64 percent for white girls and by 100 percent for black girls. About half of high school girls report that they get no vigorous exercise, compared with about one-quarter of high school boys. By the time students are in fifth grade, boys participate nearly twice as much as girls in moderate to vigorous physical activity. From age 6 to 16, boys also retain fairly constant levels of aerobic power relative to their body mass, while girls' aerobic power declines unless they participate in physical training.

Researcher Michael I. Goran and colleagues at the Universities of Alabama and Vermont repeatedly measured energy expenditures, reported physical activity, and body composition among 11 boys and 11 girls, starting at age 5 and continuing until about age 10. He found that the boys increased their average total energy expenditure at each measurement year, while the girls' average total energy expenditure declined significantly by age 10 and their reported level of physical activity fell by 50 percent between the ages of 8 and 10. The girls' food intake (adjusted for their weight), however, did not decrease. These findings suggest that girls may be biologically programmed, perhaps through the effects of sex hormones, to reduce their activity level and to store excess energy in the form of fat as they enter puberty. Such a biological tendency might have evolved as an adaptation that prepares girls' bodies for eventual childbearing, but it seems maladaptive in our modern environment. The findings on girls' activity patterns underscore the need to find strategies that will encourage girls to continue to be physically active throughout childhood and adolescence.

Sallis suggests that girls' decline in physical activity at around the time of puberty could also be socially motivated. Girls at this age worry about looking good and often become self-conscious. "As their bodies develop, they feel like the boys out there are watching them," he says. "And as girls spend more time fixing their hair, they become less interested in sweating."

🐾🐾🐾

A variety of ambitious projects have been mounted to gauge the health effects of providing kids with better, more vigorous physical education programs at school. The outcome from such studies is that children unquestionably benefit from having more and better school P.E. time, as measured by increases in their cardiovascular fitness, strength, endurance, and even academic performance. However, the track record of most such programs in preventing obesity has been disappointing. One of the most intensive P.E. programs tested so far, as part of the large, federally funded Child and Adolescent Trial for Cardiovascular Health (CATCH), failed to reduce obesity rates in children. CATCH researchers enrolled more than 5,000 third-graders from four areas of the country as participants in an ambitious three-year program to improve diet and boost activity levels. Designed primarily as an effort to reduce children's blood cholesterol levels and other heart disease risk factors, its effects were assessed in intervention schools and control schools. (The CATCH study is described in more detail in Chapter 7.)

In the P.E. component, classroom and P.E. teachers received special training on providing fun activities geared toward getting kids to spend at least 40 percent of their P.E. class time in moderate to vigorous activity. The CATCH trial succeeded admirably in getting children to play harder: kids in the intervention schools spent more than 50 percent of their P.E. class time in moderate to vigorous activity (compared with 37 percent of class time for kids in the control schools, already a respectable percentage). Kids in CATCH intervention schools also spent more time outside school hours in vigorous physical activity and made healthier food choices. Yet surprisingly, the program did not show evidence of preventing obesity. The body fat content of children in the program, as measured by BMI and skin-fold thickness, did not differ from that of children in control schools. The federally sponsored program Pathways, a similar large, school-based intervention designed specifically to reduce obesity in American Indian children in grades 3 through 5, also did not reduce BMIs.

James Sallis led a two-year California study of an intensified P.E. program called SPARK (Sports, Play and Active Recreation for Kids), in which fourth- and fifth-graders received physical education classes incorporating aerobic dance, jogging, jump rope, basketball, Frisbee, and other games intended to promote high levels of activity. Just as in the CATCH intervention, the goal in SPARK was to minimize the amount of time that any student was not moving. One group of kids took classes with P.E. specialists; one group received SPARK classes led by classroom teachers who had received special training; a third group served as the control. In both the specialist- and teacher-led groups, children in SPARK significantly increased their in-class activity levels and energy expenditures. Girls in the program showed marked improvement in two fitness measures: their time for running a mile and the number of sit-ups they could do in a minute. (Boys' fitness scores did not differ from those of the control group—perhaps because, as mentioned previously, boys already tend to be more physically active than girls at this age.) There was also some evidence that SPARK increased students' enjoyment of physical education and even enhanced their academic performance, and its P.E. program has since been widely adopted for children from preschool to middle school. But SPARK participants did not increase their activity levels outside school, nor could the study document an impact on fatness as measured by BMI or skinfold tests.

Sallis's conclusion, as he expressed it at a medical conference recently: "School P.E., no matter how good, is not going to fix the problem" of childhood obesity. In practical terms, there is simply not likely to be enough time during the regular school day for children to get all the physical activity that they need. Sallis is now focusing on finding ways to expand physical activity opportunities at other times, especially after school, which he considers the most critical time to get kids moving. "If they're not active after school, then they're not active," he says.

Still, it's worth noting that a few school-based physical activity programs have had an impact on body fat. An especially intensive P.E. program was tested on fifth-graders in seven schools in Adelaide, Australia. Ten-year-old children in an intervention group received 1 hour and 15 minutes per day of endurance training. Kids in the control group received the schools' standard 30-minute P.E. classes. At the end of 14 weeks, those in the endurance group were not only fitter but showed a significant reduction in fatness, as measured by skin-fold thickness, compared with children in the control group. The schools in the study adopted the intensive daily P.E. program, and two years later, fifth-graders in the participating schools had less body fat and a lower percentage of obesity than fifth-graders in the same schools prior to the introduction of the intensive program. Despite this positive outcome, given the heavy academic demands on today's students and teachers, few health experts or educators are optimistic about the chances of getting U.S. school systems to offer students five hours per week of intensive P.E. classes.

A California pilot program, Dance for Health, provided a small but promising field test of an "alternative" form of P.E. A Stanford medical student devised an innovative dance-based program and tested it among 81 African American and Latino children. The program, led by trained Stanford students, consisted of three 50-minute classes each week during the regular school day in which seventh-graders did dance and aerobics to hip-hop music. Children in the study were randomly divided into two groups, with one group attending the dance classes and the other attending regular P.E. classes, which also met for 50 minutes three times a week. No differences were seen among boys, but girls in the Dance for Health classes significantly lowered their BMIs and their resting heart rates compared with girls in the regular P.E. classes, indicating that they lost body fat and became fitter.

The lesson of Dance for Health was not lost on Tom Robinson, a Stanford University pediatrician who once intended to be a primary care doctor in an underserved area but who instead has devoted his career to figuring out how to get people to adopt healthier habits. After years of studying human behavior, Robinson has learned a key lesson: preaching and punishment don't work. People, especially kids, do things because they want to, not because someone has told them it's healthy. The secret is to make people want to do things that are good for them. Dance has become Robinson's stealth weapon in the battle to get kids to be more active. Hip-hop, African dance, Mexican *ballet folklorico,* Hawaiian hula, even Black Panther step chants from the 1960s—instructors are teaching all of these styles to elementary and middle school girls as part of various studies Robinson and his team are currently conducting on obesity prevention. "I've yet to find an 8- to 10-year-old girl who doesn't like to dance," he says.

A friendly man with salt-and-pepper hair and a ready smile, Robinson moves nimbly around his cluttered Palo Alto office, hopping over stacks of papers and journals piled on the floor. His own scientific publications span many of the more important preventive medicine themes of the past 20 years—smoking, exercise, alcohol abuse, seatbelt use—but in recent years he has focused almost exclusively on preventing obesity. "That has become, to me, the public health challenge of the next century and where we can make the biggest impact," he says. By testing obesity prevention programs in schools and communities, "I feel I can do more, achieve more and learn more than I could if I were only treating patients as a pediatrician."

Like a number of other researchers, Robinson has been investigating multicomponent efforts to prevent obesity: encouraging children to exercise, trying to reduce the time they spend watching television or sitting at a computer, and teaching them to make healthier food choices. Although program activities often take place at a school or community center, researchers are trying to involve parents and to influence how entire families behave. For example, the Stanford Adolescent Heart Health Program focused on tenth-graders in four ethnically diverse high schools and offered 20 lessons about diet, physical activity, and the health risks of smoking. It also taught teenagers specific skills for resisting peer pressure to smoke or adopt other unhealthy habits. Compared with students outside the program, tenth-graders in participating schools improved their diets, activity levels, and physical fitness and showed reductions in BMI and body fat.

As part of the Girls' Health Enrichment Multi-site Studies (GEMS), a federally funded study currently testing strategies to prevent obesity in African American girls, Stanford researchers and members of the local community are conducting a multipart program in Oakland, California. More than 290 girls between the ages of 8 and 10 have been recruited to Stanford GEMS, which started in 2003 and is to run for two years. Those assigned to an intervention group receive after-school classes about their cultural heritage as well as African American dance. Because African American girls have high rates of obesity and also rank high in hours of television watched per week (an established risk factor for becoming overweight), GEMS participants also get regular home visits from staff members during which they are coached and given incentives to reduce TV watching time. The program aims to maximize family and community involvement. Family members regularly flock to GEMS "jamborees" to see their girls perform. When planning such celebrations, girls and parents are urged to reconsider the role that certain foods traditionally play. "If someone asks can they bring in a cake for a birthday, we say, 'Think about whether the dance instructors can come up with a special chant instead,'" Robinson explains.

After two years, the effects of the intervention will be measured by comparing the changes in the BMIs of GEMS participants with those in a comparison group of girls who are receiving nutrition education materials and newsletters. The members of this control group also attend periodic family nights and health events, but they do not receive dance and cultural heritage classes or the TV reduction component. A parallel GEMS study, using a different intervention design, is being carried out by a research team at the University of Memphis in Tennessee.

Robinson says that girls in the Oakland program have responded enthusiastically, practicing their dances at home and eagerly helping to choose music for classes and performances. In an earlier pilot study for the program, researchers noted a reduction in girls' weight concerns, an improvement in their grades, and fewer symptoms of depression— "things that may be even more important" to the girls themselves than being overweight, Robinson notes.

GEMS and similar prevention programs currently being evaluated are complex interventions rather than simple tests of the impact of boosting children's physical activity levels. Robinson acknowledges that if GEMS is found to reduce girls' obesity risk, researchers will have to tease out the relative contributions of the dance sessions versus the television intervention or the cultural heritage classes. "We'll be able to look at the dose of each," Robinson says. "It'll give us some idea of what are the mediators of change."

🐜🐜🐜

Most of the scientific research that I've been describing has focused on trying to get kids to be physically active by making them do something specific: play harder in P.E., for example, or take a hip-hop dance class. But some of the most promising findings on preventing obesity have come from studies that asked a different question: Is it possible to reduce obesity in children simply by getting them to cut down on the time they spend being *inactive*? The answer seems to be yes—and so far, the results of such research suggest that one of the most effective things a parent can do is get children to reduce the amount of time they spend watching TV.

One of the strongest pieces of evidence supporting this strategy comes from Tom Robinson's work. In 1999 he published the results of an intervention that focused solely on television watching, a study that other researchers often cite as a landmark advance in obesity prevention. In a clinical trial involving 198 third- and fourth-grade students, he showed that simply getting kids to cut down the time they spend watching TV and playing video games—without changing anything else—reduces their chances of becoming fat. The study, published in the *Journal of the American Medical Association,* represented the first time anyone had tested the effect of reducing TV watching on obesity without at the same time trying to influence what children were eating or how much they exercised. Despite ample earlier epidemiological data that linked time spent watching television with obesity risk, many in the research community and the public were still stunned to discover that just getting kids to watch less TV seemed to help protect them from unhealthy weight gain. To Robinson, such a strategy had cried out to be tested. "It was obvious to me that somebody had to do an experiment," he recalls.

Two northern California schools participated in the study. In a randomly chosen intervention school, children in the third and fourth grades were taught a series of lessons to motivate them to reduce TV and video time to a maximum of seven hours per week, while kids in those grades at the other school served as the control group. Families of children in the intervention group received electronic television allowance meters that could be locked onto the power plug of a TV set to aid them in budgeting their kids' viewing time. The device could be set to turn off the TV when the weekly allowance was used up. Participants, families, and teachers were not told that the study's purpose was to assess the intervention's impact on obesity. At various points near the beginning and end of the eight-month study, participants from both schools were asked how much time they had spent the previous day and the previous Saturday watching television or videos and playing video games. They also reported information on their food intake, physical activity, and other sedentary behavior. At the beginning and end of the study, researchers calculated the participants' BMIs, performed other measurements to assess their body fat content, and tested their cardiovascular fitness.

As expected, children in the intervention group significantly decreased their TV viewing time (by about one-third from baseline level). They also reported meaningful decreases in video game use. This change in behavior was reflected in their bodies. Compared with children in the control group, those in the intervention group showed smaller increases in their BMIs and other measurements reflecting body fat. Although the kids in both the intervention and control groups showed an increase in BMIs and other body measurements during the school year (as is normal for growing children in this age group), the ones in the intervention group gained an average of about 2 pounds less and nearly an inch less in their waist circumferences. These effects occurred in the entire intervention group, but the impact of the intervention was greatest in children who had higher levels of body fatness at the start of the study.

Susan Yanovski, a government scientist who administers funding for obesity research at the National Institutes of Health, remembers being elated by Robinson's findings and was almost immediately inspired to put them into practice in her home.

"A couple of days after that study came out in *JAMA*, my kids announced that they had saved all their money and were about to purchase a Nintendo," she recalls. "I said, 'OK, but we're putting in a TV allowance meter.'" Yanovski's children complained at first, but now the TV meter—the same type Robinson used in his study—has become part of their lives. She sets it to give each of her three children an allowance of four hours of TV time per week. They are allowed to pool their time for a maximum of 12 hours. There's also a meter on the family computer to monitor the kids' nonhomework use.

"They budget their time like they would their allowance," Yanovski says. "If they're in the middle of a show or a game and they run out of time, it turns off. I think it's fabulous." But Yanovski adds that she has been surprised and disappointed by the reaction she gets when she tells other parents about the device. Only a couple of her friends have followed her example. "Most people say, 'That's a great idea, but my kids would never stand for it,'" she reports.

Americans of all ages spend more of their leisure time watching television than engaging in any other activity. In 1997, using data gathered by Nielsen Media Research, Robinson estimated that between the ages of 2 and 17, children in the United States spend an average of more than three years of their waking lives watching TV. Their relationship with the small screen begins early—long before they can read and, in some cases, even before they can walk or talk. In 2003 a survey of a national sample of parents conducted by the Kaiser Family Foundation revealed some startling information about infants' and toddlers' exposure to technology: two-thirds of children under the age of 2 are exposed to television, a DVD player, or a computer on a typical day, for an average of two hours. One-quarter of children in this age group have a television in their bedrooms.

As they get older, today's children rely increasingly on television and videos to fill their leisure time. Between the ages of 2 and 7, kids in the United States spend an average of 2.5 hours per day watching TV, DVDs, videotapes, or playing video games. Between the ages of 8 and 18, the average time spent in such pursuits rises to 4.5 hours per day. More than 40 percent of the third- and fourth-grade children in Robinson's California TV intervention study had a television set in their bedrooms. By the time kids are in middle school, a Boston study found, more than half sleep in a room with a TV.

The link between time spent in TV viewing and obesity rates in children and adolescents was first detected 20 years ago. In 1985 William Dietz and Steven Gortmaker identified TV watching as a risk factor for childhood obesity by analyzing data from a national health and behavior survey, and this association has since been documented repeatedly in other epidemiological studies. To be sure, most such studies have had the drawback of being cross-sectional, looking at a group of children at a particular point, rather than being prospective (assessing kids' viewing habits and monitoring the change in their BMIs over time). It's impossible to tell with certainty from cross-sectional studies

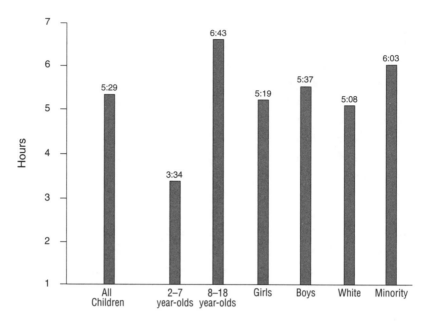

Daily media use among children, including television, video games, radios, cassette tape players, VCRs, compact disc players, and computers.
Source: See Notes.

whether a factor is a cause or a result—for instance, whether television watching makes a child overweight or whether being overweight prompts a child to watch a lot of TV.

However, a 1996 study by Gortmaker suggested that a "dose-response relationship" exists between hours of television watched and the likelihood of being overweight. And Dietz and Gortmaker's original 1985 study did contain some prospective evidence indicating that TV watching was a contributing factor to weight gain: it found that in a national sample of more than 2,000 children, those who had watched more hours of television when they were between 6 and 11 years old had higher rates of obesity later when they were between 12 and 17.

A television set in the bedroom appears to be an especially strong risk factor for kids. Barbara A. Dennison of Columbia University reported in 2002 that preschoolers with a TV set in their bedrooms were 31 percent more likely than those who did not to have BMIs above the 85th percentile for their age (the category termed "at risk of overweight" in official health guidelines). Gortmaker estimates that having a television in the bedroom automatically adds an average of an hour per day to a child's TV viewing time. "Never put a TV set in the room where a kid sleeps," he advises parents. "You sort of lose control of your kid in a whole range of ways."

It seems like common sense to assume that people who watch a lot of television are likely to be fatter than those who don't because they spend less time moving their muscles. (Such thinking is probably the logic behind the term "couch potato.") Although scientific evidence certainly supports the assumption that TV and related technologies contribute to obesity risk by making children more sedentary, this is apparently not the entire explanation. Tom Robinson notes that when TV was introduced into small communities in Canada and Scotland, children's participation in physical activities decreased. On the other hand, in Robinson's own study testing the effect of reducing kids' TV viewing time, he found, surprisingly, that children in the group who cut down on TV time did not significantly increase their levels of moderate or vigorous physical activity, nor did they become more fit. Nevertheless, they were less likely to become overweight than the control group who did not reduce their television viewing.

In addition to making kids inactive, TV watching may also influence what and how much children eat. Food and drink consumed while watching television contribute about 18 percent of the average child's total daily caloric intake on weekdays and as much as 26 percent on weekends. Some studies indicate that children eat more high-fat and high-calorie foods when they eat while watching TV, perhaps partly in response to commercials for such foods. The average child sees more than 40,000 television commercials each year. Children's programming is replete with advertising for snack foods, sweetened breakfast cereals, soda, and other foods high in fat, sugars, and total calories. Companies buy commercial time on children's shows because they know that such ads work: experiments have shown that children respond to food advertising by tending to choose and consume the advertised products. Child development research has shown that children younger than 7 or 8 do not understand that commercials are different from other program content.

Fruits, vegetables, and other unprocessed foods high in fiber and low in calories are almost never advertised, since they are difficult to brand and turn into profitable products. A 2001 study found that in families that watched television during two or more meals per day, children reported consuming significantly fewer fruits and vegetables and more red meat, pizza, sodas, and salty snacks than did children from families that did not watch TV during meals. Even the fact that many kids eat and watch television lying down may also help to boost their total food intake. A recent Australian study found that people who eat lying down take longer to feel full than those who eat sitting up, possibly because less food is retained in the stomach of a reclining person.

In addition, watching TV may consume even less energy than other sedentary activities children engage in, such as reading or drawing or talking on the telephone. In laboratory studies of kids between the ages of 8 and 12, one research group found that children's resting metabolic rates (reflecting calories burned by their bodies) were significantly lower while they watched TV than when they sat still with the television turned off. Some researchers hypothesize that kids' metabolic rates drop while watching television because they fidget less. Other scientists have failed, so far, to confirm this finding.

Tom Robinson's 1999 intervention trial on the effect of reducing TV and video time was a relatively small pilot study. He has since replicated the findings in a larger, 12-school trial; the results of that project are still being analyzed and have not yet been published. However, additional evidence supports the idea that reducing the time children spend watching TV and videos helps prevent or treat obesity. In studying obese children aged 8 to 12 in his treatment program, Leonard Epstein, a psychologist and professor of pediatrics at the State University of New York at Buffalo, found that those who were rewarded for decreasing sedentary activity lost more weight after one year than groups who were rewarded for increasing physical activity. Television watching was among the sedentary activities targeted, along with computer games, board games, talking on the telephone, and imaginative play.

Steven Gortmaker also tested the effect of targeting children's TV viewing time as part of a study of Planet Health, a comprehensive obesity prevention program for middle school children that also aimed to cut intake of high-fat foods, increase fruit and vegetable consumption, and boost kids' levels of physical activity. (Planet Health is described in more detail in Chapter 7.) Children in the schools where Planet Health was introduced significantly reduced the time they spent watching TV, and that behavior change correlated with reduced rates of obesity in the girls, although not in the boys. Gortmaker credits Planet Health's TV reduction message—absent from most other school-based obesity prevention curricula—for producing much of the program's favorable effect on children's BMIs. "My sense is that this is a very important variable that everybody has been ignoring," he says.

Similarly, researchers conducting the Growing Up Today Study, an ongoing cohort study of almost 12,000 children, found that among girls, those who increased the time they spent watching TV and videos or playing video games over a one-year period showed a corresponding increase in BMI levels. Girls and overweight boys in the study who increased their physical activity level during the same period showed a drop in BMIs. Together, these findings "all suggest that control of TV time has an impact on weight," says William Dietz of the federal Centers for Disease Control and Prevention. "The other thing about control of television time is that there's no negative. There is no adverse effect of reduced TV time." Children's TV and video time should be limited to no more than one to two hours a day, Dietz argues. That is also the official position of the American Academy of Pediatrics, which further recommends that programs watched by kids should be educational and nonviolent. The academy opposes allowing children under 2 to watch any television at all because of the activity's potential for interfering with learning to talk and play with others during a period of rapid brain development.

"Parents need to be in charge of television," Dietz says. "It's not as though that is a harmless machine in their house. If there were a guest for dinner who would make your child fat or teach them about alcohol, sex, and violence, would you actually invite [that person]? Television has that impact on children."

✿✿✿

Television and video technology are a pervasive part of American culture, and in many families they function as a cheap and convenient electronic babysitter, especially when adults are busy, stressed out, exhausted, or absent. Small wonder, then, that so many parents assume that their kids would never stand for having their TV watching time cut back. But Steven Gortmaker's research with children suggests that kids are less enamored of television than their parents might think. In testing the Planet Health program and in other studies, Gortmaker and his colleagues found that it is not difficult to persuade students in middle school and elementary school to watch less TV. "Most of the time that kids watch TV, they're not having a good time," he says. "They're just filling time—killing time."

An early lesson in the Planet Health curriculum is entitled "What Could You Do Instead of Watching TV?" The teacher explains to students that watching too much television can prevent kids from doing physical activities and can make them lose muscle strength, flexibility, and cardiovascular endurance as well as increase their risk of becoming overweight. Students make a pie chart of how they spend their time, and add up the number of hours of TV that they watch during the week. They learn that doctors recommend that they watch a total of no more than two hours of TV a day. "Watch only shows you like," the students are advised. "Take note of the times when you watch TV but aren't really interested—when you channel surf or watch reruns—and use that time to be physically active instead." Kids are asked to set goals for cutting back their TV time and replacing it with other activities. Suggestions are provided on classroom posters and on a Planet Health Web site. "They write about what else they think they can do," Gortmaker says. "They interview a grandparent about what people used to do before TV. Kids are very creative, and they can think of lots of alternatives. The key is replacing it with something they would rather be doing—and the great thing about TV is, just about anything else is more active."

Susan Yanovski suggests that parents who want to set limits on children's TV time should consider not hooking up their homes to cable television or should think about getting rid of it if they're already connected. "We don't have cable," she says. "Not only do we save the money, but there's very little on TV that our children want to watch." She also enforces a simple household rule for everyone in the family: no eating in front of the television set.

Leonard Epstein agrees that children readily find alternatives when their TV watching time is cut back. The key, he believes, is focusing on reducing the sedentary activity and letting the child choose what to do instead. He suggests that reducing the time that children spend watching TV and videos by 50 percent is a reasonable initial goal for many families. "If you just reduce access to sedentary behaviors, then kids will fill that time up," he notes. "You don't even have to talk about physical activity. They'll automatically do it." Epstein is currently using electronic TV allowance monitors successfully as part of programs both for treating and preventing childhood obesity. In one ongoing prevention study in children between the ages of 4 and 7, he says, "We're trying just to reduce TV watching and prevent excessive weight gain."

But like Yanovski, Epstein acknowledges that fundamentally changing children's relationship with television also requires changing the attitudes and behavior of the adults in the family toward the technology. So far, he has found that to be a discouragingly difficult task. "We've not had any success when we talk about getting TVs out of kids' bedrooms," he admits. "We've had absolutely no success in reducing the number of TVs in homes. We tell parents, turn the TV toward the wall, or put hard-backed chairs in front of the TV. My perception is, people just don't want to do that. They've invested the money in getting the living room just right. Now we're telling them to change, and they're not going to do it."

Steven Gortmaker finds, much to his alarm, that the majority of the parents with whom he talks are unconcerned about how much TV their children watch. "It's not on their radar screen," he says. He believes that a fundamental change in parents' attitudes will require a shift in the norms of American culture similar to the shift that has occurred in recent decades in attitudes about smoking. He tells parents: "You don't put a gun in a room where a kid sleeps. You don't put a refrigerator in a room where a kid sleeps. You don't put a TV in a room where a kid sleeps."

🐾🐾🐾

When obesity researcher Bob Kuczmarski moved with his young family to Columbia, Maryland, more than a decade ago, one of the things that attracted him to the area was the bike paths. Unlike most American suburbs, Columbia was designed as a planned community. Almost 100 miles of paved pathways for walkers and bikers connect the neighborhoods to one another, to open areas with woods, streams, and playgrounds, and to a town center with inviting shops. When the two Kuczmarski boys were small, their parents would wheel them down the path to the town center in strollers. Later the parents rode their bicycles and the boys followed along on tricycles or small bikes with training wheels. Now, at 13 and 10, the boys regularly walk or bicycle to the playground or to friends' houses. Often the whole family walks to the center, which offers sporting goods, toys, videos, crafts supplies, a Target store, and a deli. They frequently go hiking or camping together on weekends.

Life in Columbia is far from perfect, Kuczmarski admits. His property taxes are high. He commutes 30 miles each way, through heavy traffic, to and from his Bethesda office, and his wife's commute is more than twice that distance. The community, located near I-95, the highway that links Washington, D.C., and Baltimore, has its share of burglaries and drug problems. Once, Kucmarski recalls, while biking with his youngest child during the middle of the day, he came upon some teenagers on the bike path selling marijuana. Like other parents he worries about his boys' safety and does not allow them to bike or walk on the wooded paths after dark. But Kuczmarski, who grew up loving the outdoors, knows that studies have shown that the amount of time children spend outside is the strongest predictor of their overall activity level. Even though he chose an environment that offers his family the best chance he can give them of maintaining a physically active lifestyle, he wishes that he could offer his sons the same degree of freedom his parents gave him as a child in rural Ohio. "I would leave home in the summer early in the morning and as long as I was home for dinner, that's all they cared about," he says. "I was out in the woods, fishing."

Recent findings suggest that modern America's sprawling suburbs, designed in a way that forces people to rely on cars, are contributing to the obesity epidemic in children and adults. Many communities lack sidewalks and are laid out with schools and shops on the periphery, too far to make walking practical. A national study ranked the population density of 448 U.S. counties and compared the rankings with survey data on residents' weight and blood pressure. It found that people who lived in the most densely populated areas, such as New York City, weighed as much as 6 pounds less than those in the most sprawling ones. The authors speculated that the daily walking done by city dwellers made the difference. A smaller study by San Diego State University's James Sallis comparing two San Diego neighborhoods found that people living in the one close to shops and public buildings walked or biked significantly more often than those in the more sprawling neighborhood. Findings from these and similar studies are prompting policymakers and urban planners to call for changes in the way new developments are laid out and to urge "retrofitting" of some existing communities to make them more convenient, safe, and inviting for walking.

As a government researcher with the National Center for Health Statistics, Kuczmarski coauthored the landmark 1994 study that alerted doctors and the public to the existence of an obesity epidemic in U.S. adults. He later worked on other studies documenting a parallel epidemic in children. Now his job is to administer federal grants to other researchers seeking ways to combat the epidemic. Although he must spend long hours sitting at his computer, he does all he can to ensure that physical activity is part of his and his family's routine. He never takes the elevator, climbing six flights of stairs to his office each morning. Whenever he goes to the restroom, he climbs three more flights rather than use the one on his own floor. At home, he and his wife share in doing the laundry, carrying hampers up and down stairs. He mows his own lawn. His boys are required to help with housework and yardwork. He limits their television time to about half an hour a day and allows them to watch only if all their homework is done. Everyone takes turns walking the dog.

At the office, he and other experts working on obesity prevention at the National Institutes of Health sometimes trade tips about ways they have found to build a little more physical activity into their families' household routines—small things like choosing not to put in extra telephone extensions or getting rid of the TV remote control. Says colleague Susan Yanovski, "We all tend to look for ways to make things easier—but sometimes you need to look for ways to make things a little harder."

Thanks to the Kuczmarski family's active lifestyle, the boys love sports and playing outdoors. "One of their biggest frustrations is that they don't get enough physical activity at school," Kuczmarski says. Kids, he believes, have a natural tendency to maintain a balance between work and active play. "I think we sort of breed it out of our children." Research supports the view that children are happiest when physically active and suggests that parents can strongly influence their kids' chances of remaining active as they grow up. Steve Gortmaker cites research by psychologists who contacted kids as they went through their daily routines and asked them how they were feeling. Parks and recreational areas were among the places where children reported feeling best, he says. "Kids really enjoy playing and running around."

Undoubtedly, some of the influence parents exert on their kids' physical activity levels is genetic. Children of athletes are likely to inherit a variety of traits that boost their chances of being athletically talented. But parents also teach their children habits regarding physical activity by their example, by their attitudes, and by what they make available. Kids whose parents are physically active are almost six times as likely to be active themselves as are the children of inactive parents. At least one study suggests that parental activity levels are more closely correlated with exercise frequency among girls than among boys.

Parents can start early to give their children the message that moving around is both fun and valuable. Dancing around the living room with a toddler, playing catch or hide and seek, taking family walks or bike rides, making active outdoor games a regular part of holidays and celebrations—these and other simple activities help children grow up enjoying play that uses their hearts, lungs, and muscles. Early exposure to swimming, running, climbing, and ball throwing helps children acquire physical skills and confidence in their bodies, which might, in turn, lead to an increase in physical activity undertaken. Positive new experiences increase a child's self-efficacy, the sense that he or she is capable of facing a new challenge and succeeding. At the same time, play and sports should be tailored to a child's developmental level. Preschoolers, for example, can't be expected to concentrate on structured activities lasting longer than 15 or 20 minutes; most of their exercise should be free play.

Organized team sports can develop athletic skill and team loyalty but should not become a child's exclusive focus. Children also benefit from learning the skills used in individual sports—such as swimming, bicycling, tennis, running—that they may be more likely to continue to do as adults. Parents who emphasize competition, hold unrealistic expectations, and criticize a child's performance run the risk of souring their children's attitude about sports and physical activity. According to the AAP, the factors that foster a positive attitude toward sports in kids are "fun, success, variety, freedom, family participation, peer support, and enthusiastic leadership." Experiences likely to prejudice children against continuing to participate in sports are "failure, embarrassment, competition, boredom, regimentation, and injuries."

Besides encouraging physical activity at home, parents can play a vital role in advocating opportunities for kids to be active at school and in the community. Physical education is an important and often neglected component of the school curriculum. "I think we need to get parents to put pressure on the school districts to reallocate more funds away from [organized sports] and more for physical education," says James Sallis. Afternoons are a time when parents—regardless of their own schedules and where their children go after school—should try to make sure their kids have a chance to move around and burn energy, he advises. If a child does not come home after school, parents can try to ensure that active play is encouraged at the after-school program or child-care setting. They can also see that balls, jump ropes, and other sports equipment are available to kids and can link up with other families to research local sports opportunities, organize games and activities, or form carpools. "Let them be active first, either around the neighborhood or around the after-school program," Sallis recommends. "We like for kids to be active before doing homework, because they can do the homework after dark. It takes two things: it takes the community making those opportunities available, and it takes the parent taking advantage of those opportunities."

🐜🐜🐜

James O. Hill considers himself a realist: in tackling the obesity epidemic, he believes in asking people to make small changes. As director of the Center for Human Nutrition at the University of Colorado Health Sciences Center and as an expert in obesity treatment and weight management, he knows firsthand from years of research how hard it is for overweight people to keep pounds off once they've lost them. Nevertheless, he believes that slowing or stopping the obesity epidemic in children and adults could happen if a large percentage of the U.S. population would be willing to make a small, conscious, permanent change in how much they eat and how much they move each day.

Hill's research shows that among formerly overweight people who have successfully reduced their body weight, keeping the excess pounds from coming back typically requires a high level of activity—about an hour a day. "That's the one thing that's causing most of the failures out in the real world, and people don't understand that," he says. But considerably less activity—about 15 or 20 minutes a day—is sufficient to prevent weight gain from occurring in the first place. Thus, Hill reasons that the best strategy for reversing the obesity epidemic is to target the entire population and get people to modestly increase their activity levels. "I think the future is, we have to stop weight gain," he says. "If we did that, in a couple of generations we would be out of the epidemic."

That principle prompted Hill to develop Colorado on the Move, an initiative launched in his home state in 2002. The program's goal was to get Coloradans—young or old, fat or thin—to walk an additional 2,000 steps per day, which amounts to about a mile. Hill reasoned that trying to get program participants to reach 10,000 steps per day—a level of activity that health experts consider desirable for adults—was too ambitious, considering the sedentary, car-dependent lifestyles of many people. The program offered participants belt-mounted pedometers and asked them to find out how many steps they took daily and then boost that total by 2,000. It combined a media campaign with local efforts and special events in schools, workplaces, and communities. People were also given alternatives to walking through guidelines for converting other activities, such as biking or swimming, into an equivalent number of steps. Posters and advertisements provided an array of suggestions for ways to boost the daily step count: Get off the bus earlier and walk to work. Park farther from the grocery store, and always return the shopping cart to the storage area after unloading groceries. Take the stairs instead of the elevator. Take after-dinner family walks.

In surveys of participants around the state, Hill and his colleagues were able to show that people using the pedometers did increase their daily step counts—often by even more than 2,000 steps a day. Now he's trying to document the same result in a larger statewide survey and to do studies that determine whether a small daily increase in activity has a measurable impact on a population's obesity rates. Hill says that 200,000 people in Colorado have participated in the program and that at least seven other states have set up similar initiatives. A national version, America on the Move, was launched in 2003, with plans to expand to all 50 states during the next few years.

Meanwhile, James Hill is working on perhaps the biggest challenge inherent in this and similar communitywide campaigns: trying to ensure that participants continue to *maintain* their new, healthier level of activity. "If you just give people a stepcounter, they'll get excited about it for a while and then they won't do it," Hill says. "Sustainability of the program depends on giving people a continued reason to do it and to monitor their steps."

The original idea behind the Colorado on the Move program was to shift people's energy balance by getting them to adopt at least one behavior per day that eliminates 100 calories. The average American adult gains about 2 pounds a year as a result of taking in more energy (in the form of food) than is burned by resting metabolism and physical activity. For most adults, Hill calculates, weight gain can be completely avoided if people can shift their energy balance to prevent them from storing about 50 calories per day as fat. Since excess calories ingested are not stored by the body with 100 percent efficiency, he estimated that most adults could avoid gaining weight if they shifted their energy balance by about 100 calories a day, through some combination of increasing their physical activity and reducing their food intake. Walking an extra 2,000 steps daily will accomplish that goal. So will going without a chocolate chip cookie for dessert. The program's designers would prefer that participants try to do both, although counting steps with a pedometer is far easier than tightly monitoring daily food intake. People need not count their daily calories, Hill emphasizes. "Counting calories is too hard, too cumbersome. What we are doing is those two simple messages: walk 2,000 [extra] steps and eat 100 calories less."

The goals are the same for children participating in Colorado on the Move. Hill cites preliminary data indicating that the approach can prevent weight gain, at least in girls and in women. In one study, researchers enrolled families who had at least one overweight child and encouraged them to do two things: walk 2,000 extra steps each day and eat a healthful cereal for breakfast. (The latter goal was chosen because research indicates that people who eat breakfast reduce their risk of becoming overweight.) Hill said that in the family study, girls who participated in the program had lower rates of becoming overweight than girls in a control group, and mothers who participated in the program actually lost weight. No significant effects were seen in the boys or their fathers. Another study conducted in middle school students found that participating in Colorado on the Move increased children's physical activity, but Hill says he does not yet have data showing whether it reduces their BMIs.

Colorado on the Move is expanding into schools and is enrolling increasing numbers of children. Hill aims to keep the program's message simple. He adds that he chooses his battles carefully. For instance, the program does not seek to reduce TV watching because Hill does not believe it's possible to get large numbers of people to make that change. "Even though I totally think TV viewing is related to inactivity and obesity, I'm not going to expend my effort getting people to watch less TV," he says.

Many food and beverage manufacturers and fast food restaurant chains have responded to publicity about the obesity epidemic by establishing initiatives to promote physical activity, so Colorado on the Move has attracted plenty of corporate sponsors. Its national parent program, America on the Move, is sponsored primarily by food and beverage companies—Pepsico, Cargill, and Masterfoods USA, according to information provided by a link on the program's Web site. Hill says that in order to promote physical activity he is quite willing to work with companies that many people might view as contributors to the obesity epidemic. "We would be very happy to partner with McDonald's," Hill states. "Our approach is, the McDonald's of the world aren't going to go away. . . . People are going to eat at McDonald's. If they can go into McDonald's and come out having eaten 100 calories less than they would have, or with a physical activity message, then I think we've made progress."

CHAPTER 6

Programming Babies for Health—Before and After Birth

Pushing strollers festooned with tote bags and diapers, Kristen and Linda wheel their infant daughters into a sunny lounge on the seventh floor of INOVA Fairfax Hospital, a busy hospital in a Washington, D.C., suburb. Both women are first-time mothers. At the moment, neither is worrying about her child's long-term health or future risk of becoming fat. They have come to attend a weekly breastfeeding support group, and their biggest worry right now is whether their babies are getting enough to eat. Kristen's daughter, Katie, is 7 weeks old today. Kristen has been nursing her without much difficulty, but recently she and Katie seem to have hit a bump in the road. "After 15 or 20 minutes, she'll be slowing down but then she'll start kicking, arching her back, rooting around. She seems to want more," Kristen says. "She flips out. She pulls at the nipple." Katie's fussing has made Kristen wonder whether there could be a problem with her milk supply.

Linda's daughter, Grace, is only 5 days old. Lying next to plump, wide-awake Katie, she looks impossibly tiny and fragile. She was born at 38 weeks' gestation, 2 weeks before her due date—a little early, but not early enough to be considered premature. She weighs just under 6 pounds and seems to sleep all the time. Like many newborns, especially premature babies, in the days after birth she developed a relatively high blood level of a natural substance, bilirubin, formed by the chemical breakdown of a blood protein. Because her liver—responsible for removing bilirubin from the blood—is still immature, the "bili" level in her bloodstream has so far stayed somewhat high, and it's a natural sedative. Very high levels of bilirubin can damage a newborn's brain. Although Grace's levels are nowhere near that dangerous range, her pediatrician has been tracking them and will start treatment if they don't come down on their own. Poor Linda has been told by the doctor that breastfeeding every two hours will help Grace excrete the excess bilirubin, but she has to work hard to get the baby to wake up long enough to nurse. Linda looks pale, exhausted, and desperate. "She's jaundiced. She's lost a fair amount of weight," she tells Debbie Tobin, a nurse and professional lactation consultant who runs the breastfeeding support group. "I'm trying to get her enough milk to help with the jaundice and help with the weight loss. . . . Do you think that as the bili numbers go down she won't be so comatose?"

Tobin dispenses a stream of information, reassurance, and advice to both mothers. She tells Kristen that Katie's steady weight gain means her mother has an ample milk supply. Katie's behavior most likely means that the 7-week-old is developing a "flow preference": she has decided that she likes nursing better when Kristen's milk flows out rapidly, as it does first thing in the morning or at the start of a feeding, and gets impatient when the flow slows down, as it does toward the end of a feeding or at the end of the day. Kristen can speed up the flow by interrupting nursing to massage her breasts or compressing them to squeeze out more milk. "Babies figure out that nipple stimulation causes letdown" of milk, Tobin says. "Katie has her own way: pulling on the nipple. Some babies will start humming. Some will start patting. Older babies will actually push" the breast. "They'll knead, like dough."

She checks Linda's breasts and reassures her that she, too, has plenty of milk for her baby; her challenge will be finding ways to keep sleepy Grace awake and feeding. "Undress her," Tobin says. "Make a high-pitched noise. Whistle." Tobin pulls off the sleeping baby's pink gown, stripping Grace down to her diaper. She rubs the baby's chest, her back, her feet. She holds Grace against her forearms and rapidly tilts her first upside down, then right side up. Grace finally comes to and starts crying in a tiny voice that sounds like a creaky door hinge. Tobin helps Linda to position Grace on a shelf-like breastfeeding cushion that fastens around the mother with a Velcro belt. She shows her how to get the baby to "latch on" to the nipple properly so she can suck efficiently without hurting her mother. "If she falls asleep, count to 10, then whistle and jiggle her," Tobin advises.

Linda practices and takes notes. She decides to buy one of the special cushions. Kristen, with the confidence born of seven weeks' successful experience, assures her that it won't always be this hard. "Every week is different, trust me," she says. "Every day is different." Linda writes down Kristen's telephone number and struggles to recall her own. "If you [breastfeed] every two hours, you really have no downtime," she says. "You can't function on 20 minutes' sleep every two hours. . . . I'm so brain-dead I can't even remember my mobile number."

🐾🐾🐾

Developing the knowledge and skills required to be a good parent isn't easy. Faced with a newborn, a first-time mother often feels as if she's trying to interpret the cues and minister to the needs of a tiny alien. That feeling can arise even during pregnancy. Pregnant women are sometimes encouraged to think that building a baby is a lot like building a house: invest in high-quality construction materials (a wholesome diet) and let the contractor—the woman's own body—do the rest. The development of the unborn infant proceeds invisibly, through complex processes that seem beyond the mother's control. After the first few months she can feel the fetus moving around in her uterus, and as the long weeks of pregnancy creep by, she devotes herself to maximizing her baby's well-being by trying to eat healthy foods "for two" and find time to exercise her ever-heavier body.

Even the most detail-oriented mother-to-be may not realize just how much her activities during pregnancy influence her baby's development. Her food choices; her body's fat stores and her rate of weight gain; her overall health; her stress level; the faint sound of her voice transmitted through her abdominal wall; her habits regarding alcohol, tobacco, medicines, and drugs—all of these factors contribute to the fetus's internal environment. A growing body of research on a relatively new scientific subject known as fetal programming indicates that the fetus has its own system of sensors for picking up signals about what kind of world it will be born into, signals that may influence the activity of various genes, affect the pattern of overall development, even entrain the baby's future food preferences. "The new paradigm recognizes that much of the development of organ systems and programming occurs in fetal life and during the first few years of life," says Matthew W. Gillman of Harvard Medical School, who studies factors in the fetal environment that may contribute to future obesity and disease risk. Various studies suggest that the environment in the womb can affect an individual's later risk of obesity, as well as the risk of heart disease, diabetes, cancer, osteoporosis, neuropsychiatric illness, and asthma.

Before birth, an infant's future risk of obesity is linked to the health, body size, and nutrition of its mother during pregnancy. Both the woman's BMI before conception and her rate of weight gain during pregnancy contribute to her infant's growth pattern before birth and are linked to the child's future risk of obesity and of certain other medical problems. After birth, the parents' decisions about infant feeding also play a role in determining future obesity risk. Research evidence suggests that simply by breastfeeding rather than formula feeding a woman can moderately reduce her baby's chances of becoming overweight later in life. Flavors from foods that a mother eats may also be transmitted to an infant in breast milk, possibly influencing the child's eventual food preferences. Later, when the baby is introduced to an expanding array of "table foods" during the first two years of life, the foods and beverages offered to the growing child by parents, siblings, grandparents, and caregivers will help establish future eating habits. Careful choices about what and how to feed a baby or toddler can become the basis of a lifelong healthy diet.

The more researchers probe the causes of the obesity epidemic, the clearer it seems that preventing unhealthy weight gain in America's children will require adults to make profound changes in many of their own choices about diet, activity, and lifestyle.

🐾🐾🐾

In the United States, women are starting pregnancy fatter than ever before. At least 44 percent of women between the ages of 18 and 49 (considered the adult childbearing years) are overweight or obese. Rates among some minority groups are even higher—60 percent among African Americans, 62 percent among Mexican Americans. Between 1960 and the mid-1990s, the rates of obesity and overweight grew faster among women of childbearing age than among older women or among men.

An increasing percentage of women in the United States are also gaining too much weight during their pregnancies. In 2002, 21 percent of women who carried their pregnancies to term (40 weeks' gestation or more) gained more than 40 pounds, the maximum weight gain recommended by the Institute of Medicine's current guidelines. The percentage of pregnant women who gain more than 40 pounds during their pregnancies has been rising since tracking of the information began in 1989, when it was 15 percent. The large numbers of women who are either overweight to begin with or who gain unhealthy amounts of weight during pregnancy may be contributing to the rising rates of obesity evident in American children.

Both obesity and excessive weight gain during pregnancy may affect metabolic processes in a woman's body in ways that can heighten the later risk of obesity or diabetes for her child. Although the genes a baby inherits from its parents are powerful determinants of its future obesity risk, evidence indicates that environmental factors during pregnancy also have an impact. Overweight women tend to give birth to heavier babies, and infants with high birth weights (regardless of their mothers' weight status) have a somewhat increased likelihood of later becoming obese, compared with newborns who weigh less. With so many women already unhealthily heavy when they become pregnant, some experts see the potential for a vicious cycle: an epidemic of obesity that could worsen with each succeeding generation.

Overweight and obese women also have higher rates of complications than those who start pregnancy at a healthy weight. These include higher rates of diabetes and of preeclampsia, a condition causing high blood pressure and other abnormalities that can be risky for a woman and her fetus. Obese women (those with a BMI of 30 or higher) are more likely to have difficulty delivering vaginally and to need a cesarean section. They are at greater risk of such pregnancy complications as infection and postpartum hemorrhage. They have a higher frequency of stillbirth than women who are not overweight, and their infants have a higher death rate during the newborn period. Their babies also have higher rates of several types of birth defects, including spina bifida and structural heart abnormalities.

Gaining too little weight during pregnancy can also be unhealthy. Indeed, having a mother who eats too little may be more hazardous for an infant's future health than having one who eats too much. Although guidelines for healthy weight gain during pregnancy vary considerably depending on a woman's initial BMI, a minimum of about 15 pounds of weight gain is recommended even for someone who is obese when pregnancy begins. Unfortunately, the percentage of pregnant women who fail to gain even this minimum amount has also been increasing—from 9 percent in 1989 to 12 percent in 2002. If a woman fails to take in sufficient nutrients to adequately nourish her developing fetus, she may have a baby who has been partially starved before birth and as a result is at increased risk of future heart disease, high blood pressure, diabetes, and stroke. Such babies are born smaller than other full-term infants and are referred to as "small for gestational age," or SGA. Most evidence indicates that they do not grow up to have high rates of obesity. Nevertheless, many studies have found that in later life they often have an unhealthy pattern of fat distribution and an unusually high likelihood of developing the metabolic syndrome, the pattern of abnormalities associated with a high risk of diabetes, heart disease, high blood pressure, and related circulatory disorders.

"We're looking at trouble on both ends of the birth weight spectrum," says Matthew Gillman. Research findings suggest that the babies with the lowest risk of future health problems are those whose birth weight is "appropriate for gestational age," or AGA, falling somewhere in the middle of the normal range rather than at either extreme. The range of appropriate birth weights depends, of course, on whether a baby is born prematurely or at full term (37 to 42 weeks gestation). Full-term infants are considered appropriate for gestational age if their birth weight is greater than 2,500 grams (about 5.5 pounds) and lighter than about 4,000 grams (about 8.75 pounds).

Experts are increasingly urging women to try to attain as healthy a weight as possible *before* they try to become pregnant, but when pregnancy begins, weight-loss attempts should cease. Every pregnant woman should promptly seek prenatal care and should ask her doctor's advice about diet and about the range of weight gain recommended for her. With proper guidance it shouldn't be too difficult for most women to eat sensibly during pregnancy. A pregnant woman who eats a healthy diet containing a variety of foods that she enjoys is sending messages to her fetus that will help prepare the baby to adopt similar eating habits. Keeping weight gain within the range recommended by her doctor and eating healthy foods may help "program" her fetus's developing nervous system and digestive organs in ways that will allow the infant, after birth, to optimally regulate her or his own appetite, food intake, and metabolism.

🐾🐾🐾

Throughout history, midwives and physicians have recognized that when a fetus grows too slowly inside the womb, something is amiss. Too little food for the mother has historically been the commonest cause, and it remains a frequent factor today in communities where many people are poor. Yet even when food is abundant, some fetuses grow too slowly for other reasons—for example, because a pregnant woman smokes, because she is restricting her food intake in an ill-advised effort to avoid gaining weight, because she is abusing alcohol or drugs, or because there is a medical problem affecting the blood supply to the placenta, the specialized organ that provides nourishment to the fetus. Whatever the cause, the chances of survival and future health are endangered if the fetus does not receive sufficient nutrients during the critical period of development.

But an excess of nutrients during development is also bad for the fetus. Doctors first learned this lesson in the twentieth century by caring for diabetic pregnant women and their newborns. With the discovery of insulin as a diabetes treatment, it was possible for the first time for young diabetic women to remain healthy enough to have children. However, the disease makes pregnancy high risk, and pregnant women with diabetes need careful medical monitoring. A pregnant woman whose diabetes is not well controlled by insulin or other treatment sends abnormally high levels of glucose and other nutrients to her fetus through the placental circulation. Her fetus responds to this overabundant energy supply by producing high levels of its own insulin, a hormone that accelerates growth by promoting the storage of glucose and other nutrients in tissues. As a result, the fetuses of women with uncontrolled diabetes often grow very big, with an increased amount of body fat and large internal organs. These infants' size places them at heightened risk of delivery complications and injuries. They also have higher-than-average rates of intrauterine death and of birth defects.

A small percentage of women who are not diabetic before becoming pregnant develop a pregnancy-related form of the disease known as gestational diabetes. Although these women were previously making enough insulin for their own bodies' needs, pregnancy places excessive demands on the insulin-producing beta cells of the pancreas. In a woman with gestational diabetes, the pancreas can't churn out the hormone in sufficient quantities to keep the mother's blood glucose level within a desirable range. The risk of developing gestational diabetes is higher than average in women who become pregnant relatively late in their reproductive years. The risk is also higher in women who are nonwhite, those who are overweight, and those who smoke.

The body's added demand for insulin occurs because pregnancy is a time when the interplay of various hormones causes dramatic shifts in a woman's metabolism, explains Frank R. Witter, director of labor and delivery at Johns Hopkins Hospital in Baltimore. "The amount of insulin goes up, but so do the amounts of hormones that work counter to insulin," points out Witter. "Overall, the mother's blood sugar in pregnancy is lower, normally, than it is when she's not pregnant. . . . Glucose [in her bloodstream] is preferentially shunted over to the baby. The baby uses it as primary fuel." Meanwhile, the mother's metabolism "is geared up to use fats [as fuel] more than she would normally. It's a shuffling around of the fueling system so that the readily available glucose goes to the unborn child."

Gestational diabetes is usually a relatively mild form of diabetes, one that can frequently be treated with diet alone and that most often abates when pregnancy ends. Nevertheless, it poses risks for mother and infant if it is not identified and treated. Pregnant women are routinely screened with an oral glucose tolerance test. An hour after drinking a solution containing 50 grams (a little under 2 ounces) of glucose, a woman's blood glucose level is measured. If it's above a certain level, she undergoes a more extensive version of the test, with sequential measurements of blood glucose to determine whether her pancreas is producing enough insulin. If a pregnant woman is diagnosed with gestational diabetes, Witter says, she is usually given a diet aimed at preventing sudden rises in blood sugar but not necessarily designed to restrict calories or prevent weight gain. With such a diet, "the patient's limited insulin response to food intake can result in a continued good range for her blood sugar," he says.

It was by studying the long-term health of infants born to diabetic mothers that researchers became aware of the possibility that presenting too rich a feast of nutrients to a fetus might program that child for later obesity risk. Infants of diabetic mothers "are born large but decrease their weight into a normal range thereafter; however, they have a significantly increased risk for obesity by 6 to 10 years of age (50 percent prevalence)," writes pediatric endocrinologist Dennis M. Styne. Researchers at Northwestern University monitored children of diabetic mothers into adolescence and found that these children had higher rates of obesity and of impaired glucose tolerance (a prediabetic condition) than did the children of women who had not been diabetic during pregnancy. Whether the chances of future obesity are heightened in children of women who were not diabetic until they became pregnant is controversial. Some studies of infants born to women with gestational diabetes have concluded that they share the same elevated obesity risk as the infants of other diabetics; others dispute this finding.

Why blame the fetal environment at all for causing a heightened risk of obesity or diabetes in the children of diabetic women? Couldn't those risks be caused instead by genes transmitted by the mother? Some studies have tried to untangle those two possibilities. For example, in the Northwestern University studies mentioned above, researchers found that the risk of obesity and of impaired glucose tolerance in adolescents whose mothers had been diabetic correlated with high levels of insulin production by those children while in the womb. A high fetal insulin level (measured in the amniotic fluid that bathes the fetus) thus signaled a more severe impact of the mother's diabetes on the fetus—and also was linked to a greater risk that the child could become obese or diabetic years afterward. That finding provides evidence for an impact of the fetal environmental on future health that is independent of genetically transmitted risk.

The Pima Indians of Arizona, as we have seen, are both genetically and environmentally predisposed to obesity and diabetes. Studying members of this tribe has greatly aided scientific understanding of how genes and environment interact. Researchers found Pima families in which the mothers had been diabetic during pregnancies with some of their children but not during others. Studying these Pima children when they were between the ages of 9 and 24, researchers found that those who had been exposed to diabetes before birth had a higher frequency of obesity than their unexposed siblings, even though the sibling pairs shared many of the same genes. "This tends to isolate the fetal environment as a potentially important period," says Matthew Gillman.

Screening women for diabetes is a recommended part of routine care during pregnancy. By making sure that all women get timely prenatal care, including diabetes testing and proper treatment for gestational diabetes, it should be possible to reduce the chances of later obesity in infants of diabetic mothers. Still, the impact of the fetal environment on the obesity epidemic doesn't seem to be limited to children of women with diabetes. Bigger babies, whatever the reason for their large size, appear to be at higher risk in later life of becoming overweight. More than two dozen studies have examined the association between infants' birth weight and their BMI as children or adults. Almost all have found a direct association: "Higher birth weight is associated with higher attained BMI," notes Gillman.

Once again, it's difficult to tease apart the influence of genes from that of environmental factors in the womb. We know that overweight parents are genetically predisposed to have children with a higher-than-average likelihood of becoming overweight. But Gillman points out that a child's risk of being overweight is more closely associated with obesity in its mother than in its father. Although this finding could imply sex-linked transmission of certain genes that influence obesity risk (for example, genes located on the X chromosome, which children of both sexes receive from their mothers), it also suggests a possible role for the prenatal environment. Gillman and colleagues studied the relationship between birth weight and later obesity rates in more than 14,000 young adolescents, aged 9 to 14, who were the sons and daughters of women participating in Harvard's ongoing Nurses' Health Study of behavioral factors and disease risk. They found a correlation between birth weight and later obesity risk. Average birth weight was about 3.5 kilograms, or 7.5 pounds. Each additional kilogram (2.2 pounds) of weight at birth above this average figure increased an infant's risk of being overweight during early adolescence by about 50 percent. (For instance, the risk of adolescent obesity was 50 percent greater for a newborn weighing 5.7 kilograms [12.5 pounds] than for an average-weight infant.) Part of that correlation was related to whether the mother was overweight or obese. When the researchers performed a statistical adjustment to take into account the mother's BMI, the association between high birth weight and later obesity risk was reduced but not eliminated.

Why does being big at birth—sometimes called "large for gestational age," or LGA—apparently increase a person's chances of becoming overweight later on? How could factors that prompt a fetus to grow rapidly in the womb somehow "program" that same individual to store extra pounds as fat during childhood or adulthood? One possibility, supported by some studies, is that whatever leads to rapid growth in the womb produces an infant with a higher percentage of body fat than an average-sized newborn. LGA babies have relatively higher levels of body fat and a lower percentage of lean body mass than babies whose weight is appropriate for gestational age. Having a larger number of fat cells, or bigger fat cells, at birth may predispose an individual to later weight gain.

Another theory suggests that exposure to certain environmental factors during fetal life—for instance, high levels of certain nutrients or of specific hormones, such as insulin or leptin, the hormone made by fat cells discussed in Chapter 2—somehow presets the fetus's future metabolism in a way that encourages energy storage. Some research in animals supports this notion: newborn rats fed a high-carbohydrate diet respond by producing excessive amounts of insulin even as adults and become obese. Recent studies implicate leptin as a key player during fetal and infant brain development, influencing the wiring of connections among the nerve cells of the arcuate nucleus of the hypothalamus, a brain area that regulates feeding and body weight. A natural surge in leptin levels occurs in mice during the first week of life and in human fetuses before birth. Oregon researchers found that in newborn mice that are genetically lacking in leptin the hormone surge does not occur and nerve cell connections within the arcuate nucleus do not form properly. When researchers treated such baby mice with leptin timed to mimic the natural surge, nerve cells in the arcuate nucleus responded by growing branches and forming normal-appearing connections. The leptin surge had to occur during a critical period in early life; giving leptin later did not have the same effect. "Nutritional or other environmental factors that suppress leptin during brain development may have lasting effects on an individual's ability to regulate body weight," suggested Richard B. Simerly of Oregon Health and Science University, one of the authors of the study.

The quantity and mix of nutrients a fetus gets before birth—or receives as an infant during the newborn period—may lastingly influence the development or function of specialized nerve cells in the areas of the hypothalamus that regulate appetite and metabolism. The findings of German researcher Andreas Plagemann imply that an excess of nutrients, either during fetal life or during early infancy, might influence a person's lifelong regulation of food intake or energy expenditure. In rats that were "overfed" from birth by being raised in unusually small litters, Plagemann and colleagues were able to demonstrate persistent differences in nerve cell activity and in production of chemical messengers within the appetite-regulating areas of the hypothalamus, and these differences were associated with overeating and obesity in the animals as adults.

We have seen that babies who are especially large at birth have an increased likelihood of later becoming overweight or obese. But what about babies who are especially small, although not premature? The outlook for such infants seems puzzling. If they are not at risk of obesity, why do they nonetheless seem to be at risk of many of the medical problems we think of as being associated with obesity: heart disease, diabetes, stroke, high blood pressure, and the metabolic syndrome? The answer is not yet clear, but several decades of research have provided a partial explanation. It seems likely that SGA babies, who grow poorly before birth, often grow up to develop these diseases not because they are vulnerable to obesity but for other reasons. Most evidence suggests that they are not at heightened risk of becoming overweight: indeed, they tend to maintain a lower-than-average weight for their height throughout childhood and into young adulthood. But the body fat they do store is more likely to be distributed in an unhealthy pattern than the body fat of people whose weight was average at birth. They are prone to central or abdominal obesity, a pattern in which fat is disproportionately stored on the abdomen or trunk rather than the hips or limbs. As I explained in Chapter 1, this type of fat distribution has undesirable effects on metabolism. A tendency to store fat around the abdominal organs is associated with a heightened risk of the metabolic syndrome and an increased likelihood of developing diabetes and heart disease.

It is not known why SGA babies are more likely than others to develop this pattern of fat distribution. Neither is it clear whether their tendency toward abdominal fat storage is the entire explanation for their vulnerability to the metabolic syndrome and diseases related to it. A related theory holds that undernutrition during fetal life alters the development of the fetus's pancreas, especially the beta cells that make insulin, affecting the way the body processes glucose and other nutrients. Undernutrition may also affect later patterns of secretion of cortisol, a "stress hormone" that influences metabolism and fat distribution. In addition, SGA babies tend to be born with relatively small kidneys, and their kidneys remain on the small side, since this crucial organ grows its full complement of functioning cells during fetal life. Some experts believe that subtle differences in kidney function may help explain why people who were SGA infants are later at greater risk of high blood pressure.

The effects of undernutrition on a fetus may even vary according to the period of pregnancy during which the developing fetus lacks sufficient nutrients. Almost 30 years ago, in the famous "Dutch famine" study, researchers observed that young Dutch men whose mothers had been exposed to wartime famine during the early weeks of their pregnancies were more likely than other men to be overweight as adults. However, men whose mothers had suffered famine in mid-to-late pregnancy were more likely to have the pattern of central obesity and metabolic abnormalities common to SGA babies. Although experts today say that certain aspects of the Dutch study's design may have reduced the validity of its findings, it provided some of the earliest suggestive evidence of a possible impact of the fetal environment on later health.

David Barker, a British researcher who has searched extensively for possible links between prenatal factors and disease in later life, explains in his book, *The Best Start in Life,* that a developing fetus sets an overall growth trajectory early in pregnancy, based on the level of nutrients being delivered via the placenta. If the nutrient supply is low throughout pregnancy, a fetus grows slowly and develops into an infant who is small all over. But a fetus can also to some degree alter the trajectory during pregnancy in response to changes. If the nutrient supply starts out adequate but falls off at some point in middle to late pregnancy, brain growth may be preserved at the expense of the growth of kidneys, liver, muscle, or fat stores. Thus, although two infants may be born with identical birth weights, their body shapes, pattern of growth in the womb, and perhaps many other aspects of their development may be quite different.

During the 1950s, says physician Frank Witter, obstetricians were determined to limit pregnant women's total weight gain in order to prevent them from having big babies. Larger babies posed a greater risk of complicated deliveries and more often needed to be delivered by cesarean section. But by being overly strict about weight gain, Witter says, doctors unknowingly contributed to a crop of SGA babies who grew up to face an elevated risk of heart disease, diabetes, and other disorders: "Regrettably, that's what we did. With some of our recommendations in the '50s, we were starving women to lower the birth weight." Some doctors even encouraged pregnant women to smoke, he recalls, reasoning that it would reduce their food intake and keep their babies small. In the 1950s, pregnant women were commonly advised to try to limit weight gain to 20 pounds. "That was more than someone who was heavy should have gained, and less than somebody who was underweight should have gained, and we probably produced some of the problems with central obesity and metabolic syndrome by restricting weight gain," Witter observes. He adds: "Many people are invested in 'Big baby, big problem. Little baby, all safe.' In fact, as we're looking at them longer and longer, both have problems that are of a different nature. The baby who's at the least risk for obesity is the child who is appropriate for gestational age in weight."

🐾🐾🐾

So far, it's unclear from U.S. birth weight statistics what impact the obesity epidemic among American women is having on the size of newborns. As women in America have become more overweight, the frequency of diabetes during pregnancy has increased sharply. About 3.3 percent of U.S. women develop gestational diabetes during pregnancy, according to 2002 figures—a 40 percent increase since 1989. It's difficult to quantify the health impacts on newborns. Fortunately, the number of very large ("macrosomic") babies, those weighing at least 4,000 grams (about 8 pounds 13 ounces) has actually fallen slightly since the 1980s, perhaps reflecting improvements in screening and prenatal care for diabetic mothers. Just under 10 percent of infants weighed 4,000 grams or more in 2000. Babies in this weight class are at increased risk for complications during delivery, including birth injuries and asphyxia.

The mean birth weight for a "singleton" baby (not a twin or triplet) born in the United States in 2002 was 3,332 grams, about 7 pounds 5 ounces. Mean singleton birth weight has remained almost constant since 1990, according to government data. In the same period the total number of low-birth-weight infants has increased, but this is primarily because fertility treatments have resulted in more multiple births. Babies who are small because they share the uterus with a sibling are biologically different in some respects from SGA babies who are singletons. Researchers do not have enough evidence yet to know whether some infants who are part of multiple births face similar health risks.

Interpreting small changes in infant birth weights over time is complicated, because the average birth weight in the United States is affected by whether the frequency of premature births has changed, and even by whether more full-term infants are being delivered after 39 weeks of pregnancy, as opposed to after 40 or 41 weeks. Michael Kramer, a pediatric researcher at Montreal's McGill University, has analyzed the pattern of birth weight change in Canada in ways that shed light on what may be happening in the United States. There, too, women are starting pregnancy fatter and are gaining more weight during pregnancy. Rates of diabetes during pregnancy have also increased. But an additional important factor influences birth weights in both countries: as a result of public awareness of the risks of smoking, the number of women who smoke during pregnancy has declined dramatically. In the United States, for example, the proportion fell from almost 20 percent in 1989 to 11 percent in 2002. That's excellent news. Kramer's analysis shows that in Canada the decline in smoking during pregnancy has been largely responsible for a heartening drop in the number of babies who are born small for gestational age. Eating appropriately and not smoking are the two most important things a pregnant woman can do to prevent her infant from being born SGA.

In Canada the decline in smoking, coupled with the obesity epidemic among women and the increasing frequency of gestational diabetes, contributed to a rise in mean birth weight of about 50 grams (a little under 2 ounces) between 1981 and 1997. The proportion of infants who are large for gestational age has also increased. The data suggest that in Canada "the size of babies at any gestational age is going up," Kramer says—and this shift toward heavier birth weights may be adding fuel to the epidemic of obesity there. A similar upward trend in birth weights has not been documented in the United States, but some experts worry that it could be on the horizon.

In addition to not smoking, what can a woman do before and during pregnancy to help ensure the best health outlook for her baby? "Getting yourself in the best physical shape, eating well, and getting appropriate rest—those are things that a woman can do," says Witter.

At best, that effort should get under way well before pregnancy begins. "I talk with all of my patients about their BMI," says Joan Loveland, an obstetrician-gynecologist who practices in Chevy Chase, Maryland, a suburb of Washington, D.C. For women whose BMI is over 25, placing them in the overweight category, "I tell them that their exercise program and the nutritional changes that they make are like [taking] blood pressure medication or insulin," Loveland says. Such behavioral changes are part of the prescription for having the healthiest possible baby. "What's amazing to me is that many physicians don't bring this up, because they're afraid they will offend their patients and the patients won't come back."

Ideally, any woman who is contemplating pregnancy should schedule a preconception visit with an obstetrician to go over her health history and talk about nutrition and other lifestyle factors such as smoking, alcohol use, and exercise. If she smokes, now is the time to quit. All women of childbearing age should take a daily multivitamin containing 400 micrograms of folic acid, even if they are not intending to become pregnant, because research has shown that adequate levels of this vitamin, if present at conception and throughout early pregnancy, can prevent spina bifida and anencephaly, which are serious birth defects involving the nervous system. If a woman is overweight, she can maximize the chances of good health for herself and her baby by trying to get as close as she can to a desirable BMI before she starts trying to become pregnant. Despite the fact that almost half of nonpregnant women in the United States report that they're trying to lose weight, research shows that they aren't using the strategy most likely to be effective: a combination of limiting calorie intake and increasing physical activity.

Loveland wishes that more of her patients would make a point of coming to see her for routine preconception health counseling. "Women who are seriously considering pregnancy soon, they're very motivated" to make healthy lifestyle changes, she says. "Gestational diabetes and weight gain during pregnancy really do correlate" with future health risks for the fetus. "That's a pretty compelling argument for trying to get people fit before they become pregnant." Once a woman begins trying to conceive, she should not be on a highly restrictive or unbalanced diet. Her meals and snacks should be healthy, with plenty of fruits and vegetables, fiber and calcium-containing foods (such as dairy products), and she should take a prenatal vitamin daily. She should continue to get regular exercise throughout pregnancy, unless her doctor limits her activity for health reasons. If a woman is especially anxious about the weight gain and changes in body shape that are inevitable with pregnancy, she should be sure to share her fears with her doctor, midwife, or other health care provider.

Recommendations for how much weight to gain during pregnancy should be individually tailored, depending on a woman's BMI at the start of pregnancy. Current recommendations are based on a large body of evidence indicating that adequate weight gain during pregnancy is very important for fetal growth, while excessive weight gain is associated with an increased risk of pregnancy complications and of having a high-birth-weight (LGA) infant. Generally, the Institute of Medicine and other specialty medical organizations recommend a weight gain of 25 to 35 pounds for women of "normal" weight (defined by IOM prepregnancy guidelines as a BMI between 19.8 and 26.0). Underweight women (BMI below 19.8) should aim to gain 28 to 40 pounds. Overweight women (BMI between 26.1 and 29.0) should aim to gain 15 to 25 pounds, and women with a BMI greater than 29.0 should aim to gain about 15 pounds. Every pregnant woman should talk about her own range of desirable weight gain with her obstetrician at her first prenatal visit. At each prenatal visit, she and the doctor or midwife should track her weight and discuss how she is doing.

Women should keep in mind that staying within the weight gain guidelines is not a guarantee that an infant will grow optimally, since pregnancy complications, birth defects, or various problems with fetal development may affect the pattern of growth regardless of the mother's diet and other habits. At the same time, many infants are carried to term and born healthy, at a weight appropriate for their gestational age, even though their mothers may have gained too much or too little weight during pregnancy.

Also, many pregnancies are unplanned, so it is not always possible for a woman to prepare herself in advance. But every woman, regardless of her weight at the start of her pregnancy, can do a great deal by eating sensibly, by not smoking, and by getting regular physical activity to give her baby the best possible start before birth.

🐞🐞🐞

Kristen, who attended the breastfeeding support group with healthy 7-week-old Katie, says she knew even at the beginning of her pregnancy that she planned to breastfeed. Her friends had done it, and they encouraged her. Her doctor gave her pamphlets to read. When Katie was born, she told the nurse in the delivery room, "I know you're supposed to breastfeed within half an hour [of birth]. She got me set up and told me how to do it," Kristen recalls. "I was kind of nervous about it: is this going to work? But once you get the hang of it, you get a lot better."

Katie is thriving, growing and developing beautifully, and Kristen knows her breast milk benefits her baby in numerous ways. She even playfully scolds Katie when the milk flows too fast and the baby lets some drool out. "I'm like, 'Don't drool it. That's valuable milk,'" Kristen says. "I'm going to breastfeed this child as long as I possibly can. I would like to say at least six or eight months—that would be my goal."

Breastfeeding has many proven advantages over formula feeding. Breastfed babies are less likely than formula-fed infants to have ear infections, allergies, vomiting, diarrhea, pneumonia, bronchitis, meningitis, and wheezing. They may also be less vulnerable to sudden infant death syndrome (SIDS). Breastfeeding helps the mother, too: it makes it easier for her to get back to her prepregnancy weight, helps the uterus to recover from pregnancy, reduces her risk of breast and ovarian cancer, and may even improve bone strength and reduce her risk of hip fractures after menopause. And breastfeeding enhances the bond between mother and infants. For all these reasons, the American Academy of Pediatrics recommends breastfeeding, preferably exclusively, until an infant is at least 4 to 6 months old.

"Women sometimes say to me, 'Isn't formula just as good as breast milk? Won't my baby do just as well on formula?'" says lactation consultant Debbie Tobin. "I can't in good conscience tell a woman that formula is just as good as breast milk because it would be lying, based on the research."

Many new mothers don't realize that a woman who breastfeeds is probably also giving her baby a degree of protection against future obesity. Of all the various strategies for preventing childhood obesity that have been investigated so far, the scientific evidence supporting a protective role for breastfeeding is "the most compelling," in the opinion of pediatric obesity expert William Dietz. Based on research results, Dietz has estimated that universal breastfeeding could prevent about 15 to 20 percent of the obesity cases that currently develop in children before the age of puberty. Although research on this topic has produced a somewhat mixed verdict, a number of recent large studies suggest that breastfeeding provides an infant with at least a moderate reduction in the risk of future obesity.

Choosing whether to breastfeed a newborn—and how long to continue—are personal decisions highly influenced by a mother's social, cultural, and economic circumstances. Mothers of newborns need education, encouragement, and social support in order to adopt and stay with this method of feeding. Many new mothers are relatively uninformed about how to breastfeed or how to solve problems they may experience with nursing. Many belong to families or cultures in which breastfeeding has not been widely practiced recently, so their own mothers or other relatives can offer little help. Women often need to return to work quickly in order to support their families and find it difficult to adjust their schedules, job demands, and child-care arrangements in order to keep nursing.

Fortunately for children in the United States, breastfeeding has come back into vogue in recent years. In 2001, according to a national survey, almost two-thirds of children under the age of 3 had been breastfed at least as newborns, compared with only 54 percent a decade earlier. Still, most women don't nurse their babies as long as is recommended by health guidelines. At 6 months of age, only 27 percent of babies were still nursing, and at 1 year only about 12 percent were still receiving any breast milk. These figures lag behind national health goals set by the federal government, which specify that by 2010 the proportion of mothers breastfeeding their infants should rise to 75 percent in the newborn period, 50 percent at 6 months, and 25 percent at 1 year. Despite the AAP's recommendations, exclusive breastfeeding declines sharply after the first few months of life: only 8 percent of U.S. infants are being exclusively breastfed by the time they are 6 months old.

For various reasons it has been difficult for scientists to determine whether breastfeeding has an impact on later obesity risk. A major one is that women who breastfeed are more likely than those who do not to be white, thin, well educated, and relatively well off. All these characteristics are also associated with having children with lower rates of obesity. Among racial and ethnic groups in the United States, breastfeeding rates are lowest in African Americans, who also have among the highest rates of obesity. In addition, overweight women in general have more difficulty breastfeeding than slender women, so they are less likely to initiate nursing and more likely to discontinue it.

Correlating breastfeeding and future obesity risk is not a straightforward process. The links between breastfeeding and various other characteristics are considered by scientists to be potential "confounding factors," which means that such factors may misleadingly influence their results. For example, if a study shows that children who were breastfed as infants have lower BMIs than children who were fed infant formula, it could simply be because the mothers of the formula-fed children were fatter and transmitted a genetic vulnerability to obesity—not because of the way their infants were fed. Moreover, most studies on this topic have been retrospective, or "looking backward": researchers have assessed the BMIs of a group of children at a particular age and have then depended on parents' memories to categorize how those children were fed as infants. This kind of study design is considered less accurate and informative than a prospective study, in which children are recruited as infants and then monitored as they grow.

A few years ago nutrition researcher Nancy F. Butte of Baylor College of Medicine reviewed evidence from studies published up to 1999 and determined that most (about a dozen) had found "an insignificant effect" of breastfeeding on later obesity. Only four studies suggested that breastfeeding provided some protection, and Butte concluded that confounding factors (other differences between mothers who chose to breastfeed and those who chose to formula feed) may have been responsible for the apparent benefit. However, Kathryn G. Dewey, a professor of nutrition at the University of California at Davis, recently assessed a group of larger and newer studies and reached a different conclusion. Dewey reviewed 11 studies, 9 of which were too recent to have been considered by Butte. All met certain criteria, such as size: they had to include at least 100 children in each comparison group. She also looked for studies in which children were at least 3 years old when researchers assessed their weight status, reasoning that breastfeeding's impact on obesity risk might become more evident in older children. And she sought studies in which researchers had adjusted the design and statistical analysis to try to tease apart the influence of breastfeeding from other potentially confounding factors.

Of the five studies on children aged 3 to 6 that Dewey considered, three found that breastfeeding reduced later risk of overweight. Of the six studies on older children and adolescents, all but one found evidence of a protective effect of breastfeeding. In four of these, this effect persisted after researchers statistically adjusted for the most important potential confounding factor, the mother's BMI. Several studies also used statistical techniques to control for other potential confounders, such as socioeconomic status, maternal smoking, parents' level of education, children's diets and physical activity levels, and additional factors. Among studies suggesting a protective effect, Dewey found that the odds of becoming overweight were about 21 to 34 percent lower in children who had been breastfed than in those who had been formula fed. "Although the effect of breastfeeding may not be large, its role in preventing child overweight could still be of significance" given the breadth and severity of the obesity epidemic currently facing the United States, she concluded. The finding of clearer results in older children also suggested that the beneficial effects of breastfeeding on obesity risk are delayed. "Breastfeeding may have a 'programming effect' that does not manifest itself fully until the preadolescent and adolescent growth spurt occurs," writes Dewey.

How might breastfeeding an infant affect that child's body size later in childhood? One frequently proposed explanation is that a baby who breastfeeds has much greater control over his or her calorie ingestion, which allows the infant's body to become better at regulating its own energy intake. Research findings indicate that nursing babies do manage their own intake; for example, babies whose mothers produce higher-fat breast milk generally consume less than the infants of mothers with lower-fat breast milk, Dewey posits. Formula-fed infants, in contrast, are often encouraged by the parent or caregiver feeding them to consume a specified amount of formula, even after the baby shows signs of losing interest in the bottle. Formula-fed babies consume more calories and gain weight faster than breastfed infants. Formula-fed babies "may be modestly overfed," says William Dietz. "With my own children, when we shifted them to a bottle, I know that I tended to look at the bottle toward the end of the feeding. It's easy to push a couple of extra swallows."

As I mentioned earlier, evidence from animal studies indicates that overfeeding in the newborn period is correlated with increased numbers of fat cells, higher insulin levels, and differences in the development of brain regions that regulate food intake. In humans as in animals, overfeeding during infancy might have a lasting effect on brain development, metabolic hormones, and future regulation of body weight, suggests Nicholas Stettler, a pediatric nutrition specialist at the University of Pennsylvania. Stettler and colleagues showed in a study of more than 19,000 U.S. children that rapid weight gain during the first four months of life was associated with a higher risk of being overweight at the age of 7. In another study of 300 young African Americans in Philadelphia, Stettler and other researchers showed that rapid weight gain in the early months of infancy was associated with a doubling of obesity risk at age 20. Although some infants are probably genetically predisposed to rapid weight gain, it's possible that overconsumption of calories during a critical period of early life might also program a baby for later obesity risk. "You cannot really overfeed a breastfed infant. Whereas with a formula-fed infant, the mother can potentially override the appetite of the child," Stettler says. "The hypothesis is that if they learn to rely on outside cues rather than their inner cues, maybe that is learned behavior that is leading them, in the long term, to rely more on the environment rather than on their appetite."

The higher levels of calories and protein ingested by formula-fed babies also result in higher levels of insulin, a hormone that stimulates fat deposition, in the infants' bloodstream. Among Pima Indian children, who as we have seen are genetically, as well as environmentally, predisposed to obesity, one study found that those who had been breastfed were less likely to be overweight or to have diabetes than those who had been formula fed. Hormones or other unidentified substances present in breast milk could also play a role. For example, breastfeeding may help program the developing infant's response to leptin, the appetite-regulating hormone produced by fat cells, either through direct exposure to leptin in breast milk or by other mechanisms.

The only scientifically definitive way to find out whether a behavior (such as breastfeeding) causes a certain outcome (such as reducing obesity) is to conduct what's called a randomized controlled trial: recruit a large cohort of pregnant women, randomly divide them into two groups similar in racial, ethnic, and socioeconomic makeup, and assign the women in one group to breastfeed and those in the other group to formula feed their infants. But such an experiment would be unethical because breastfeeding is already known to be superior to formula feeding for other reasons. However, an ongoing European trial may be the next best thing. Known as the PROBIT trial, it enrolled more than 17,000 women and their infants in the Republic of Belarus during 1996 and 1997. All of the mothers participating in the trial intended to breastfeed. Women randomly assigned to one group received an experimental intervention aimed at promoting and supporting breastfeeding; women assigned to a second group received standard medical care. Throughout the 12-month period, women in the intervention group were significantly more likely to continue breastfeeding than those in the control group. Researchers are continuing to monitor the health and BMIs of the children, and Stettler is hopeful that future data from the PROBIT trial may help answer the question of whether breastfeeding really helps protect against later obesity.

In the meantime, what recommendations for mothers and infants can be made, based on research so far? As pediatricians "we recommend breastfeeding for at least four months and possibly exclusively for six months," says Stettler. "That's really the only safe recommendation we can make so far. I wouldn't make the recommendation, with formula-fed infants, to restrict their intake until we know whether the association we've shown [between formula feeding and a possibly higher risk of later obesity] is explained by underlying genetic factors or whether there are other causal relationships."

Women who are planning to breastfeed should ask their obstetricians to check their breasts and nipples during pregnancy. Certain conditions, such as nipples that are inverted or retracted, sometimes make nursing more difficult, but steps can be taken to improve such factors. Many hospitals also offer a breastfeeding class for pregnant women as part of their childbirth and parenting education programs. Most also offer breastfeeding classes and individual coaching for new mothers while they are in the hospital after childbirth. A new mother should take advantage of such opportunities to get all the instruction and support she can before taking her baby home.

AAP guidelines recommend that breastfeeding should begin as soon as possible after birth and that newborn infants should "room in" with their mothers rather than being kept in a nursery. Newborns should be nursed whenever they show signs of hunger and initially will need to feed 8 to 12 times every 24 hours. The guidelines also recommend formal evaluation by a trained observer of how well breastfeeding is going before a mother and her infant are discharged from the hospital and again in the early days at home. Breastfed infants, according to the guidelines, should not be given other fluids as supplements unless there is a medical reason for it. Supplements and pacifiers should be avoided if possible, or at least until breastfeeding is well established. "Exclusive breastfeeding is ideal nutrition and sufficient to support optimal growth and development for approximately the first six months after birth," the guidelines state. Breastfed infants under 6 months old generally do not need water, juice, or other foods.

Some medical experts argue that the health benefits of breastfeeding are already so well established that there is no point in spending additional research funds to try to quantify breastfeeding's benefits in preventing obesity, which may turn out to be modest compared to the impact of changing other behaviors that are fueling the epidemic. A recent exchange at a medical conference between Michael

Kramer of McGill and Matthew Gillman of Harvard illustrates the debate on this point. Arguing that breastfeeding probably plays a minor role in obesity protection, Kramer said, "If you had everybody in the United States exclusively breastfeeding for six months . . . we would still have an obesity epidemic in this country." Gillman said he agreed. But, he added, "Just think how much the increase in obesity would be worse if we hadn't seen the increase in breastfeeding over the last 20 years!"

🐜🐜🐜

Breastfeeding may have yet another benefit for babies, according to the surprising results of research by Julie A. Mennella, a scientist at the Monell Chemical Senses Center in Philadelphia. Mennella studies the role of early experiences in the development of food and flavor preferences during infancy and childhood. Her findings provide fascinating evidence of how clearly certain smells and tastes are perceived by very young infants. Mennella's work and that of some other scientists suggests that certain foods impart a perceptible flavor to breast milk and even to the fluid that surrounds the fetus before birth, thereby providing the fetus and the breastfeeding infant with a foretaste of foods that are important parts of the mother's diet, foods that are prepared and served in that infant's family and culture. Such findings suggest that food exposures during early infancy and even before birth may help program a child's eventual dietary likes and dislikes. "Breast milk is almost like a flavor bridge from what the infant experienced in the womb to the foods at the table," Mennella says.

In evolutionary terms, taste and smell are the oldest senses, linked to deep, primitive areas of the brain. For animals and humans, the proper functioning of these senses contributes to survival, since they help an individual seek out and eat foods that are safe sources of energy and reject others that are potentially dangerous or poisonous. "These senses are well developed in utero," Mennella says. "However, the infant and child are living in their own sensory world." Because the senses of taste and smell continue to develop as a child grows, babies and children apparently perceive some smells and flavors more strongly than adults and others less strongly.

Taste refers to the sensory experience that occurs when chemicals stimulate the taste receptors, specialized groups of cells distributed on the tongue and in other parts of the mouth and throat. Each of the five types of receptors detects a different taste: sweet, salty, sour, bitter, and umami (or glutamic acid, a natural substance found in such foods as asparagus, cheese, meat, tomatoes, and *kombu,* a type of seaweed used in traditional Japanese cuisine that researchers employed to identify the source of the distinctive umami taste).

Smell or olfaction is a separate sense caused by chemical stimulation of olfactory receptors, structures located on a small area of tissue in the nasal cavity. Hundreds and perhaps thousands of odors can be detected by humans, thanks to the existence of a huge number of unique receptor proteins. The flavor of a food or beverage depends on a combination of its smell and taste. While the primary taste of a food may be salty or sweet, its odor is what allows the person eating it to make fine flavor distinctions, such as being able to tell whether a piece of fruit is a strawberry or raspberry, or whether an ice cream is vanilla or chocolate. Smell's key contribution to our perception of flavors explains why foods taste flat to us when we have a cold.

Taste buds are well developed by the midpoint of pregnancy, and there is some evidence that fetuses can detect sweet, sour, and bitter. Newborn infants will relax their faces and suck when offered a sugar solution and will grimace and even stick out their tongues when given a solution containing citric acid (sour) or quinine (bitter). Infants' preference for sweet-tasting liquid is an adaptive trait, since human breast milk is noticeably sweet. In contrast, the ability to taste salt does not develop until about 4 to 6 months of age, and perceptions of salt and bitter continue to change during infancy and childhood.

Although an individual's basic taste preferences are probably partly determined by genes, there is evidence that early experiences, even before birth, can modify them. For example, college students whose mothers had suffered frequent morning sickness during pregnancy (and who, as a result, probably spent part of their pregnancies mildly depleted of water and salt) showed a stronger preference for salty foods than students whose mothers had not had morning sickness. In general, children prefer saltier foods than adults, but experience with salty foods in childhood tends to strengthen an individual's liking of salt.

Taste is not the only sense that develops before birth. Newborn infants are sensitive to a variety of odors and respond with changes in facial expression, body movements, and heart and breathing rate. An infant can recognize her or his mother by smell alone, and breast-fed infants can distinguish a breast pad worn by their mothers from pads worn by other lactating women. If certain foods, such as garlic or spices, are eaten by a pregnant woman, their odors permeate the amniotic fluid that bathes the fetus. Animal research suggests that foods to which a fetus is exposed in this way may be preferred by the infant after birth.

The foods a mother eats also flavor her breast milk. Garlic, anise, carrot, mint, blue cheese, vanilla, and undoubtedly many other substances can be detected by a breastfeeding infant. Babies even seem to enjoy some of this variety. Mennella and a colleague, Gary Beauchamp, showed that breast-fed infants stayed attached to the nipple longer after their mothers had eaten garlic or vanilla than after their mothers had eaten bland foods. "The flavor varies with the time of day and with what the mother is eating," notes Mennella. She theorizes that this physiological flavoring of breast milk may serve an adaptive function. Since the infant already recognizes and enjoys the underlying taste of the milk, faintly flavored breast milk may promote the baby's acceptance of certain foods later on. She points out, for example, that babies are quicker to accept infant cereal if it is prepared using their mothers' milk. Commercially produced infant formula, in contrast, always tastes the same. It does not expose a baby to new flavors.

In an intriguing test of this theory, Mennella and colleagues conducted a study in which pregnant women who intended to breastfeed their babies were assigned to one of three groups. One group drank carrot juice regularly during the last part of pregnancy; a second group drank carrot juice regularly during the first two months of breastfeeding; a third group (the control group) avoided carrot juice and drank water. When the babies were old enough to be introduced to solid food, their reactions to carrot-flavored cereal versus plain cereal were videotaped and analyzed. Those who had been exposed to the flavor of carrot juice either before birth (in amniotic fluid) or as infants (in breast milk) were less likely to grimace in response to carrot-flavored cereal than were babies in the control group, and they were rated by their mothers as enjoying the carrot-flavored cereal more than plain cereal. A study by another pair of researchers found that breast-fed babies more readily accepted a new vegetable than did formula-fed ones. Mennella suggests that this willingness could be due to their having tasted the specific flavor of the vegetable in breast milk, to the fact that they were simply more used to tasting a variety of flavors, or both.

The idea that flavors in breast milk might educate a baby's palate and help establish lifelong food preferences gives breastfeeding a layer of significance beyond its established health benefits. "Odors and flavors that have acquired meaning early in life have long-lasting responses," says Mennella. "These senses can be trained. They are a reward system that encourages us to seek out pleasurable sensations. They underlie the strength of preferences for foods and eating habits."

🐘🐘🐘

During their first two years of life, babies and toddlers make the transition from getting their nourishment from breast milk or infant formula to eating "table foods" like the rest of the family. Their early experiences with food are vital to the development of dietary preferences and eating habits that are likely to persist, at least to some extent, throughout their lives. Ample evidence exists showing that many U.S. families are not doing nearly enough to make sure that their infants or toddlers are learning to eat a healthy diet during this critical time. The Feeding Infants and Toddlers Study (FITS), a recent national survey sponsored by the Gerber Products Company, found that as toddlers in the United States approach their second birthday, their diets start to look more and more like the unhealthy, highly processed, calorie-dense diets of older children and adults. Their intake of yellow vegetables like carrots and squash drops dramatically. French fries become the "vegetable" they most often consume. One-third of them eat no fruit on a typical day, but one-quarter drink soda or a sugar-sweetened beverage. Says Barbara Devaney, a policy researcher who participated in the FITS survey, "We may not be able to affect what infants and toddlers are eating without addressing what older children and adults are eating."

When the time comes to introduce a baby to solid foods, how should parents handle this important and exciting period in their child's development? What can they do to promote good health and encourage lifelong healthy eating habits? To begin with, they should not start solid foods too soon. Infants younger than about 4 months old lack the mouth and tongue coordination needed to swallow solids, and could choke even on infant cereal, which has traditionally been the first solid food a baby is offered. In addition, there is evidence that too early an exposure to foods other than breast milk or infant formula increases a baby's risk of developing food allergies. Some studies have even suggested that babies given infant cereal before the age of 3 months may have an increased likelihood of producing antibodies (chemicals made by the immune system) against the beta cells of the pancreas. Such antibodies may be involved in causing damage to these insulin-producing cells, increasing an individual's risk of developing type 1 diabetes.

Many new mothers are urged by relatives and friends to give their babies cereal when the infants are as young as a few weeks old, in the mistaken belief that it will satisfy the baby's appetite better than breast milk or formula and make the baby sleep through the night. Such beliefs are well intentioned but misguided. Solid foods do not improve the diet of very young infants or make them sleep better. In the 1980s Cleveland researchers scientifically studied the question of whether putting cereal in babies' bottles can make healthy young infants sleep through the night. Of a total of 106 infants, they randomly assigned half to a group that began receiving rice cereal at bedtime (1 tablespoon per ounce in a bottle) at 5 weeks of age, and the others to a group that received the bedtime cereal at 4 months old. A parent or other caregiver then recorded each baby's sleep pattern during one 24-hour period each week, from the ages of 4 weeks to 21 weeks. Sleeping through the night was defined as sleeping at least eight consecutive hours with the majority of that time occurring between midnight and 6 a.m. There was no statistically significant difference in sleep patterns or sleep duration between the two groups, nor was there any consistent trend.

Babies do not need solid food before the age of 6 months; breast milk or formula fulfills their nutritional needs. The earliest age that cereal introduction can ever be considered appropriate, according to feeding guidelines, is at 4 months old. The American Academy of Pediatrics recommends exclusive breastfeeding, if possible, for the first 6 months of life and gradual introduction of solid foods between the ages of 6 months and 1 year old. (If a mother decides to stop breastfeeding before her infant is 6 months old, the baby should receive only formula until the age of 6 months.) Fruit juice is also not recommended for infants younger than 6 months old.

Vegetables and fruits are traditionally the first foods to which babies are introduced after infant cereal. Pureed vegetables and soft or pureed fruits (either prepared at home or bought as commercial baby food) are nutritious and full of vitamins. As we already know, vegetables and fruits are pillars of a healthy diet for children and adults. Pediatricians often recommend introducing one new vegetable or fruit at a time and offering it for several days in a row. Part of the reason for this approach is that babies—as well as toddlers and some older children—are often slow to accept a new food, a response known as "neophobia," or fear of the new. On the first try a baby may take a mouthful, twist his face into an expression of apparent disgust, and stick out his tongue, letting the green bean paste drip gently down his chin. This doesn't mean the baby will never again eat green beans. "Really, you expect children, when they taste something strange, to kind of screw up their faces," says William Dietz. "Parents often mistake the child's expression of experiencing a novel food as an expression of dislike. Absolutely, repeated introductions do help a child get used to food."

"Probably because ingesting new substances is a risky business, most new foods are not immediately accepted," writes psychologist Leann Birch of Pennsylvania State University. A distrustful attitude toward new foods on the part of children may even be a trait that was favored during human evolution, because it was advantageous to survival. Repeatedly exposing a child to a food, however, eventually leads to acceptance in many cases. Children are also more likely to accept a food if they see family members or other children eating it. Birch found that preschool-age children who initially disliked certain vegetables began eating them after they saw other children eat them in a childcare setting. Young children in certain cultures learn to accept even spicy, "hot" foods after they see family members eating and enjoying them.

As I mentioned previously, young children's preferences for sweet and salty foods do not have to be learned. A preference for high-fat, calorie-dense foods such as pizza or French fries is apparently not innate, but research has shown that children quickly become conditioned to prefer these types of foods, probably because they're filling and rapidly satisfy hunger. In one study children were given repeated opportunities to eat soup and yogurt. Some versions of these foods were higher in fat or carbohydrates than others, hence more calorie dense, and their flavors also differed. Although children in the study initially liked the lower-calorie and higher-calorie soups and yogurts equally well, after repeated exposures they became conditioned to prefer the higher-calorie versions, especially when they were hungry.

Young children do vary individually in their liking of high-fat foods. In one study of 3- to 5-year-olds, Birch and a colleague found that youngsters who most strongly preferred high-fat foods also tended to be the fattest in the group and to have parents with the highest BMIs. It's unclear whether these children's preference was genetically based or whether it was influenced by exposure to high-fat foods in the home—or perhaps by environmental factors during life in the uterus.

Birch says that for parents of young children the take-home message of much of this research is that they need to focus on giving their babies and toddlers plenty of opportunities to eat and experience healthy foods, especially fresh vegetables, fruits, and whole grain products. Such foods form the foundation of almost all widely accepted schemes for healthy eating. "Kids don't have to learn to like sweet and salty," she says. "But if they are not offered a variety of things from the bottom of the Food Guide Pyramid," such as fresh vegetables, whole grain foods, and fresh fruits, they won't necessarily learn to like those foods. "Parents should work to get those things into the diet, rather than restricting it to foods that the child is programmed to like and accept."

This does not mean that parents should try to force a baby or toddler to eat a certain vegetable. That's a recipe for failure. British researcher Jane Wardle suggests playing a "tasting game" in which the parent gives the child the tiniest possible piece of the food that is being tried. The child can taste it and then may decide whether to eat it or spit it out. Wardle says research with families using this playful approach has shown that it helps persuade toddlers and young children to try and accept new foods.

It may be a good idea to get a baby accustomed to a varied diet. In one study, Julie Mennella and a colleague assessed several different strategies for introducing 5-month-old, formula-fed babies to carrots. All the infants were given carrots for the first time on day 1 of the study. On days 2 through 10, one group ate pureed potatoes, a second group ate carrots, and a third group, the variety group, ate one of three different vegetables—peas, potatoes, or squash. On day 11, when all the babies were given carrots, the carrots were eaten with equal enthusiasm by the all-carrot group and by the variety group. Group 1, the potato group, was less likely to accept them. Mennella also found that the variety group was the most willing to accept a new food (chicken) and that giving babies some fruit each day enhanced their willingness to accept carrots. This latter finding tends to disprove the belief, common in some communities, that if infants are given fruits at the same time as vegetables, their preference for the sweet fruits will make them more likely to reject the vegetables. Perhaps experience with variety makes babies less likely to fear and reject what is new. Summarizing her findings, Mennella writes, "Early experience with a diversity of flavors may have led to an increased readiness to accept unfamiliar flavors."

Researchers who have studied various parental feeding styles suggest that mealtimes should be an occasion for positive, cheerful interaction between parents (or caregivers) and babies. A baby should not be left alone with a propped bottle or fed by a distracted adult who does not talk to it or make eye contact. Babies and toddlers should be allowed to refuse to eat a certain food, and they should be the ones who decide when to stop eating. Parents should never use foods as bribes or rewards, nor should they withhold them as punishments. Actively and repeatedly urging a young child to eat a certain food ("Come on, Tommy, eat your broccoli!") is likely to backfire.

At the same time parents must be in charge of what a baby is offered, and all the presented foods should be healthy and developmentally appropriate for the age of the child. Just because a baby reaches for a hot dog or a candy bar does not mean she should have one! The findings of the Gerber FITS survey suggest that many U.S. parents are regularly feeding babies and toddlers highly processed sweet and salty foods. More than 60 percent of 12-month-olds whose parents were surveyed for the study were being fed dessert or candy at least once a day, and 16 percent ate a salty snack. By the age of 15 months, 30 to 40 percent were drinking sugary fruit drinks daily. Daily fare that contains high levels of sugar and salt is likely to reinforce young children's innate liking for those tastes and may discourage the development of preferences for healthy foods.

Although 100 percent fruit juice is preferable to fruit drinks because it is rich in vitamins, minerals, and nutrients, it is high in sugars and not as good a fiber source as a piece of fresh fruit. Too much fruit juice may encourage a preference for sweet beverages as a thirst quencher instead of water. The American Academy of Pediatrics suggests limiting juice consumption to 6 ounces a day for children aged 1 to 6 years and no more than 12 ounces a day for those aged 7 to 18.

At a recent medical conference, Jane Wardle contrasted the child-feeding styles of parents in France and the United States, suggesting that cultural differences in how children learn about food may be one reason why the French have much lower rates of obesity than Americans do. Citing research by social historian Peter N. Stearns, she noted that in France the emphasis is on training the appetite and teaching children to learn to eat the foods adults eat. In French families, fussy eaters are generally not allowed to demand substitute foods; instead, if children do not like what is on the menu, they go hungry until the next meal. In the United States, Wardle observes, parents are more concerned with pleasing children and worry more about whether they are getting enough to eat. Snacks are much more commonly offered than in France, and family food choices tend to be child centered. Wardle suggests that American parents might do well to adopt a more typically French attitude in teaching their young children how to eat. "We are responding to the child's instincts," she says, "but on the other hand, we are the environment that entrains the child's instincts."

CHAPTER 7

Eating Lessons at School

I n the broccoli bed the tall, gangly stalks are topped with yellow flowers. They have passed their tasty prime and are going to seed. A group of sixth-grade students are carefully pulling them out of the ground while other children follow with pitchforks, turning over the black topsoil.

"Hey, there's a snail and a baby snail," says one child.

"Oh, there's a whole bunch of snails!" cries another. A few kids squeal and back away.

A boy holds up his gloved hand. "Ew, look! This one's stickin' to my finger!"

Nearby, the garden's hens, Ella, Couscous, and Henrietta, are patrolling the vegetable and flower beds, looking for bugs. In one bed lettuce seedlings have put forth small green leaves. In another the tendrils of young pea plants are climbing up strings. A few tiny pods are already visible. The radish bed is full of bushy, vigorous-looking plants, and the leeks have sprouted skinny green stalks.

Over in the raspberry patch other sixth-graders are raking and weeding the paths between bunches of 2-foot-tall, healthy raspberry canes growing in raised beds.

"Make the path deeper than the raspberries," a boy instructs his coworkers.

On a table set up near the garden wall, seven kids are making pizza to bake in a tall outdoor oven hand built of stone and brick. On a breadboard they roll out a ball of whole wheat dough into a big thin pie, then ease it onto a large wooden paddle called a peel and paint it with olive oil. Toppings, including fresh vegetables and herbs from the garden, are set out in bowls: sautéed chard and leeks, feta cheese, fresh rosemary, and cilantro. The garden teacher, Amanda Rieux, and assistant Lissa Duerr, an Americorps volunteer, are overseeing the pizza-making process.

"David, Manta, have you seen the cilantro growing in the garden?" Rieux asks. "I'll show you where it is. Do you know what these are? These are leeks."

"We don't have to put chard on," suggests one boy. "I don't like chard."

"I want some," says another.

"You can decide as a group if you want chard," says Duerr.

The students take an informal poll. Chard lovers predominate. They sprinkle some on.

One of the teachers arrived at school several hours ago to fire up the wood-burning oven. "Do you know how hot it gets?" asks Duerr. "'Round about 650 degrees!"

With Duerr's help, David slides in the pizza. The kids wait impatiently, sniffing the aroma of fresh bread and savory vegetables that wafts through the cool spring air.

Out comes the pizza at last. They count 30 seconds to let it cool, then cut it into slices and dig in.

"Thank you, Lissa!" they murmur, between bites.

"You're very welcome. How is it?"

"Great!"

For these sixth-grade students, it's all part of an ordinary morning's lessons in the Edible Schoolyard, an acre of urban garden behind Martin Luther King Middle School in Berkeley, California. Spectacularly situated on a hill overlooking San Francisco Bay, the garden took root from the dreams of a nationally famous local chef, Alice Waters, and a visionary public school principal, Neil Smith. In the years since its inception in 1995, the Edible Schoolyard Project has become considerably more than just a garden. Through the efforts of a dedicated staff of teachers and volunteers, and with the help of aggressive fundraising and community support, it has transformed the culture of a resource-poor junior high school by creating an extraordinary learning environment. The garden and its adjoining kitchen are unconventional classrooms where the middle school's teachers integrate learning about biology, nutrition, horticulture, environmental education, cooking, and group cooperation into everyday lessons on diverse subjects, including math, science, social studies, art, drama, and English as a second language (ESL). More than 600 children spend 90 minutes of class time per week in the garden or kitchen. Sixth-, seventh-, and eighth-grade students grow, prepare, and eat their own fruits and vegetables, and kids who rarely sit down to family dinners at home get the chance to cook, set the table, and enjoy a meal together.

In the spacious, brightly painted kitchen, sixth-graders start their cooking lessons by making fruit salad, learning to use knives safely. While studying the origins of agriculture in Mesopotamia, they grow and grind grains—wheat, millet, barley, amaranth, quinoa, blue corn, flax—and bake flatbread with the flour they've made. By the time students reach seventh grade they've become skilled cooks. They eagerly compete on teams in the Iron Chef, a contest in which they are given a set of ingredients and must create a hot dish and a cold dish for a panel of adult judges in 45 minutes.

"It's very fun in here," says kitchen teacher Esther Cook. "It's really important to me that they have fun—that they not think of cooking as a potential job, but as something people do every day for the people they love. We don't out and out teach nutrition. If we can get kids to know what to eat and when, the nutrition piece is a big part of that. Parents say their kids are now interested in food. They know the vegetables, the greens, the taste of the different apples. A fair amount of what we do in the kitchen is just tasting."

New school traditions have grown up around the kitchen and garden. At the beginning of each school year, children in the school's ESL classes prepare a special dinner for their parents. During the week when children take state-required standardized tests, the staff and their student helpers produce a home-cooked breakfast daily for the entire school community. In spring the seventh-graders, whose time in the garden is ending, plant a crop of corn for the incoming sixth-grade class. The following fall the sixth-graders harvest the crop and feast on grilled corn. The lesson of that tradition, says garden teacher Kelsey Siegel, is that "you're not going to necessarily always eat what you plant."

On a bulletin board in the kitchen, teachers have pinned up a selection of "Edible Schoolyard Famous Quotes" uttered by kids while working in the garden or kitchen:

"I've never been full of vegetables before."

"I'm thankful for photosynthesis and laughter."

"Hey, look at the Golden Gate Bridge. It looks like a giant bra!"

In the universe of school gardens, Berkeley's Edible Schoolyard Project is a bright star—large, luxuriant, generously staffed, and boasting a $400,000 annual budget raised chiefly from nonprofit organizations. Yet it serves a school with a diverse student population, including many children from poor families, and it grew out of the determined work of local community activists. In those respects it is far from unique. School gardens and greenhouses, student-run fruit and vegetable stands, and farm-to-school programs have taken shape in many localities around the country, funded by local jurisdictions, nonprofit organizations, and state and federal governments. There is evidence to support the idea that such projects can influence kids' eating habits: for example, children who are involved in growing food in school gardens have been shown to increase their liking for certain vegetables. Such projects represent just one of the approaches being taken by school officials, activist groups, parents, and communities to change the way schools teach children about food and healthy eating.

Like chef Alice Waters, many people have come to believe that the food and drink children receive at school teaches them silent but powerful lessons, lessons that may leave a more lasting imprint on their minds and bodies than what they hear from teachers in health or nutrition classes. As is true of the campaign to incorporate more movement and exercise into the school day, efforts to change the school menu take various forms but share an underlying philosophy: in order to teach children to make healthy lifestyle choices, the "hidden curriculum" about food and physical activity in schools must be consistent with the overt curriculum in the classroom. Right now, the hidden nutrition curriculum in many U.S. schools is all about fast food lunch choices, high-fat chips and snacks, bake sales that feature doughnuts and brownies, and a steady supply of soda and sugary drinks from vending machines. Although this kind of school menu may resemble the diet of many families in the United States, it is teaching or reinforcing unhealthy eating habits for our children.

Schools are mirrors of our society. As such, they often displease us and make us angry. Because schools take responsibility for children, parents, educators, and other concerned adults expect them to be the best possible environments: healthier, safer, more rational, more moral, and more compassionate than other settings. When schools turn out to have many of the same flaws that exist elsewhere in America, we are outraged, yet we're looking at our own reflection.

But schools are also social laboratories. Throughout our country's history they've been experimental settings where educators and reformers have tried to solve society's problems. Public schools are the places where the majority of U.S. children over the age of 5 spend most of their waking hours. Reaching children at school is one of the most efficient ways of communicating directly with families. And because children are eager to learn and are open to new experiences and ideas, they can be effective agents of change within families. Tens of thousands of Americans probably have been motivated to quit smoking because a child or grandchild urged them to do so.

During the past few decades Americans have greatly expanded their expectations of what schools can and should provide. Schools in many places have assumed increasing responsibility for aspects of children's lives that go beyond academics, including health care, psychological counseling, crime prevention, after-school care, and even child care for the infants and toddlers of high school students. More recently the pendulum has begun to swing back toward a more academic focus. State and local jurisdictions and the federal government have moved to enforce academic standards by annual testing of students—and to penalize teachers and schools with scores that fall short. This trend has placed pressure on school systems to cut back on other priorities and to focus more exclusively on grooming students for standardized tests as official performance measures. Considering schools' pivotal position in the lives of children and families, it's not surprising that they're being asked to become important players in the nation's response to the childhood obesity epidemic.

Researchers, activists, and parents trying to combat the obesity epidemic through schools are using three major approaches. One is to improve and expand physical education programs or to find additional ways of incorporating physical activity into the school day. (Some of these efforts were discussed in Chapter 5.) A second strategy is to stop schools from selling foods and beverages high in calories and low in nutrients and to try to ensure that all the meals, snacks, and drinks available in schools are healthy. A third approach is to get schools to adopt curricula that teach the importance of a good diet and daily physical activity, curricula that also impart practical skills such as reading food labels and measuring portion sizes and that motivate students to try out and adopt new habits, such as eating more fruits and vegetables or reducing their weekly TV time.

It seems obvious that any serious and honest attempt to create a healthier school environment should incorporate all three approaches. If schools pay lip service in health classes to the importance of a proper diet yet sell sodas and junk food in vending machines, children learn the lesson that good nutrition is not an authentic priority. A similar message is transmitted if teachers extol the virtues of exercise but students rarely have P.E. or opportunities for vigorous play. Being consistent and avoiding hypocrisy are as critical to effective teaching as they are to effective parenting. Our schools must "walk the walk."

The first lunch period is about to begin at Fairhill Elementary School, in north Philadelphia. Five students from the sixth, seventh, and eighth grades have been hard at work since midmorning, carefully putting fresh grapes, strawberries, and pieces of pineapple and melon into plastic cups to make individual portions of fruit salad. Now four sixth-graders, chosen by their teachers to be this week's sellers, are carrying cardboard cartons containing fruit salad cups, paper bags, and bananas to the big plastic "fruit stand" in a hallway outside the cafeteria. As they lug their boxes across a rain-washed courtyard, they pass a large red and white truck emblazoned with the familiar Coke logo, which is parked beside the school. A Coca-Cola deliveryman is inside the cafeteria, restocking the vending machines.

The children unpack their wares at the fruit stand and write the prices—$1.25 for a small salad cup, $2.00 for a large one—on a little blackboard. Each fruit salad comes with a banana and, this week, a free "veggie baby," a small stuffed toy. Judith and Amanda will be delivering prepaid salads to teachers in their classrooms. Robin and Giuseppe will be selling salads at the stand. Being selected to make or sell fruit salads is a coveted privilege, bestowed on students who work hard and behave well. At Fairhill, which serves a low-income neighborhood whose residents are mostly Hispanic and African American, all the kids who work in the program during the year receive a share of any profits earned.

Dan Lewis, who supervises Fairhill's student-run fruit stand each Wednesday, issues instructions to Robin and Giuseppe. "The customer is going to come up and say what kind of salad they want," he tells them. "Place the salad on the counter. Give them a bag. Let them know they are getting a free veggie baby with their purchase. Only one of you should deal with the money." Lewis works for the Food Trust, a Philadelphia-based nonprofit that has received nutrition education funding from the U.S. Department of Agriculture to operate school markets, farmers' markets, and other programs designed to improve nutrition in low-income neighborhoods. Although the major goal of the fruit stand is to boost fruit and vegetable consumption among Fairhill's students, the school's food service staff would not allow it to be set up in the cafeteria. Lewis says they worried that it would take away business from the school lunch program, another federally funded program under which the USDA subsidizes the school for providing free or reduced-price meals for low-income children.

Inside the spacious cafeteria, the walls echo with the laughter and chatter of hundreds of students eating lunch. Out here in the corridor, few children pass the fruit stand. Robin and Giuseppe make most of their sales to adults: a police officer, several teachers, a man visiting the principal's office. Two cafeteria workers wearing aprons come by, eye the fruit salads, and promise that they'll be back later. "Traffic is slower here. [Students] don't walk by" on the way to the cafeteria, says Lewis. "We get a lot of chance sales—people picking up their kids, the UPS man. If there is any part that we could do better with, it would be to get more kids [buying]." Giuseppe unpacks his own lunch: a bag of chips and a large soda. Watching him, Lewis shakes his head ruefully. "There are some corner stores near every school that we [the Food Trust staff] work at," he says. "They buy chips and soda on their way to school."

Finally, business picks up. Jenny and Eduardo, two of the students who helped assemble the fruit salad cups show up with about a dozen other kids from the sixth, seventh, and eighth grades. A line forms. Robin enthusiastically hands out fruit salads and veggie babies while Giuseppe collects money. When lunch period is over Robin and Giuseppe tally the day's sales: 31 large salads, 21 small ones. Judith and Amanda return from delivering their prepaid orders. They remove a pile of cash and their order list from a manila envelope and count the money.

"Only one quarter off," Judith says. "We have $25.00 and it's supposed to be $24.75." A teacher had told her to keep the change. She smiles. "I'm so proud of myself!"

As the lunch scene at Fairhill illustrates, the nutritional environment in our nation's schools is both complicated and inconsistent. The kinds of food and drink a public school offers depend on choices made by school officials, such as the principal and the food service manager, but also on policies set at the school district level and laws or regulations passed by the local, state, and federal government. The USDA has detailed rules specifying nutritional standards for the daily school lunch (and often breakfast) served in the cafeteria, meals that are subsidized in most schools by a national government program. But the federal government does not have authority to regulate any additional a la carte items sold in the school's cafeteria, nor can it specify what kinds of snacks or drinks may be sold in vending machines or in the student store. State and city governments often do regulate some of those items, though, and in recent years impassioned battles have erupted in many jurisdictions over whether laws should be passed to eliminate vending machines altogether or to prohibit them from dispensing sodas and certain other kinds of snacks and beverages.

Of course parents also influence what's eaten at school, by making or buying children's lunches and by bringing or sending in food for special occasions. In some communities they have also become players who influence their local schools' lunch and snack menus. Clubs, teams, and organizations (such as Girl Scout troops) often sell snacks, sweets, or beverages to raise money. Teachers sometimes plan the menu for a special event, and some misguided ones use food in the classroom as a reward or incentive.

Most schools in the United States have no comprehensive nutrition policy specifying what kinds of food and drink are considered healthy or appropriate to be sold on their premises. The federal government does recommend that schools set such policies: in fact, detailed guidelines were published by the federal Centers for Disease Control and Prevention in 1996. Because few schools have accepted that challenge, the list of foods and beverages sold in most American middle and high schools is a hodgepodge. It typically includes dozens of calorie-dense snacks and drinks, foods that are often high in fat, sugar, and salt but low in vitamins and other nutrients. These items are sold to students not because they are nutritionally valuable but because they can make money for the school or its activities. Elementary school offerings tend to be somewhat healthier but still include high-fat cookies, crackers, and salty snacks.

The National School Lunch Program administered by the USDA has considerable influence on what children eat at school. Founded in 1946 with the laudable goal of fighting hunger, it has, ironically, become a target for reform by activists trying to reduce childhood obesity. The program provides free or reduced-price lunches on every school day to about 28 million children who qualify because their family's income falls below a specified level. (In 2004 a child living in a family of four with an income below about $34,000 qualified for a subsidized lunch; a child from a family of four with an income below about $24,000 qualified for a free lunch.) An almost equal number of children purchase the same cafeteria lunch at full price, typically between $1.25 and $2.50, depending on the school and the region.

The USDA sets nutritional requirements for school lunches, specifying their total calorie content, the maximum percentage of calories that should be derived from fat, and how much protein, calcium, iron, and vitamins A and C they should provide. It's up to school food service directors to plan menus that meet those requirements. The USDA subsidizes participating schools' lunch programs at a cost of more than $6 billion a year, paying the school food service a specified amount for each free or reduced-price meal served. Besides payments to schools, it also purchases certain foods from U.S. producers as a form of agricultural subsidy and provides them free to school food services, where they make up about 17 percent of the food served. Thus, the USDA's requirements and its food subsidies to the school lunch program influence what school cafeterias serve to everyone.

Critics, including some nutritionists and dietitians, charge that the dual goals of the Department of Agriculture's school lunch program—feeding children and subsidizing farmers—are often at odds with each other. For decades beef, pork, and dairy producers have successfully lobbied Agriculture Department officials to include large quantities of meat and dairy products among the foods that the program buys and donates to schools. Some details of the law governing the program even seem designed to put food producers' interests ahead of nutritional concerns. Schools are required to offer whole milk as an alternative to lower-fat milks each year as long as more than 1 percent of students opted for whole milk during the preceding year—although whole milk is high in fat and not recommended for children over 2 years old. Since school food service directors operate on tight budgets and must strive to break even each year, the types of food they can get free from the federal government are a key factor in their decisions about what goes on the lunch menu. It is also cheaper, both for food services and for the government, to use frozen, canned, and processed foods in school lunches than to purchase fresh fruits and vegetables that might spoil and have to be discarded.

Despite the USDA guidelines specifying nutritional content, most school lunches contain a higher percentage of fat than the maximum specified by government requirements. Among schools surveyed during 1998–1999, school lunches averaged about 34 percent of calories from fat. Average fat content of school lunches had declined from 38 percent in the early 1990s but remained higher than the 30 percent maximum specified by the USDA's requirements—and more than three-quarters of U.S. elementary and secondary schools had not succeeded in cutting enough fat to reach the 30 percent goal. In addition, the average elementary school lunch was providing about 10 percent more calories than what's recommended by the USDA. Salt content in elementary and high school lunches was also much higher than the maximum level recommended. States are responsible for monitoring and enforcing their school districts' adherence to the nutrition guidelines, but schools are not usually individually penalized for failing to meet the standards. It is extremely rare for a school to lose its eligibility to participate in the federal school lunch program.

In public schools I visited while researching this book, students told me the most frequent lunch entrees in their cafeterias included pizza, hamburgers with cheese, chicken nuggets, hot dogs, burritos, and macaroni and cheese. One overweight student at a District of Columbia high school said wistfully that she wished her school cafeteria would offer salad every day. "We had mashed potatoes three days in a row this week," she complained.

One of the most disheartening aspects of the lunchtime fare provided at thousands of schools across the United States is that it often seems chosen to reinforce a taste for fast food and for foods high in fat and processed carbohydrates rather than to encourage healthier eating habits. School officials sometimes contend that they are forced to serve high-fat lunch entrees like cheeseburgers and hot dogs because that is the only kind of food students will eat. But researchers have found that many students do choose lower-fat alternatives, especially if they are first introduced to the lower-fat foods or if they and their parents are informed about the health benefits of reducing fat intake. Researcher Robert Whitaker found that about 30 percent of elementary school students spontaneously chose lower-fat menu items when they were offered at lunch, and the figure rose to 36 percent after a letter went home informing parents of the low-fat lunch choices. In another study, students in some classrooms at an elementary school in upstate New York learned about the history and nutritional value of plant-based foods such as greens, black-eyed peas, and bulgur, as well as cooking and tasting such foods as part of their study of different cultures. Students in other classrooms, the control group, did not receive such lessons. When these foods were offered in the school cafeteria, students who had learned about them in class ate from 3 to 20 times more of them than did the students in the control group. "Kids like knowing about good foods that are good to eat," says obesity prevention researcher Steven Gortmaker. "Kids are looking for stuff that is different and better."

School officials in some health-conscious districts have successfully lowered the fat content in school lunches and breakfasts. For example, in Rocky Boy's, Montana, tribal leaders on the Chippewa Cree reservation worked with a dietitian to revamp the school menu in an effort to combat high rates of obesity and diabetes among American Indian children there. Dietitian Tracy Burns got rid of premade pizzas and sugary cereals. She persuaded the school bakers to switch from white to whole wheat flour. She eliminated 2 percent milk as an option (instead offering only 1 percent), instituted a daily salad bar, and increased schools' purchases of fresh fruits and vegetables. She asked school cooks to mix the higher-fat ground beef provided by the USDA subsidy with leaner ground beef or buffalo meat that the food service purchased locally. And students were no longer allowed seconds at meals except for fruits and vegetables.

The USDA has responded to concerns about the foods it provides to the national school lunch program by increasing the amount of fruits and vegetables it supplies to schools, although most are frozen or canned. The department does supply some fresh fruits and vegetables (about 21 percent of all fruits and vegetables it provides to schools), chiefly as part of a joint program with the Department of Defense, which trucks them to schools in 38 states. The USDA conducted a successful pilot program in several states that showed that offering children free fruits and vegetables as snacks significantly boosted their daily intake from that food group and shifted their diet away from candy and high-fat snacks, but the future of such programs will depend on whether government funding is made available.

Even when the main school lunch offering of the day is healthy, many students still end up eating high-fat snacks, sweets, and soda for lunch because most schools offer such items as a la carte choices in the cafeteria, the school store, or vending machines. Schools throughout the United States opt to balance their budgets and fund activities by selling a bewildering variety of snacks and beverages, often in direct competition with the regular school lunch. Students may pick such items because they prefer them or because their lunch break is short and the line for the regular lunch is too long.

Although a federal law prohibits foods of "minimal nutritional value" from being offered in school cafeterias during mealtimes, the only items that fall into that category are soft drinks, gum, and certain candies. Many other foods—pizza slices, brownies, layer cake, French fries—supply enough nutrients to be legally sold as competitive items, even though they are high in sugar or fat. And federal law allows vending machines to dispense candy and soda throughout the school day, as long as the machines are not located in the food service area.

In a USDA-funded study of 2,300 school districts, more than 80 percent of middle schools and high schools sold a la carte items. Vivian Pilant, director of school food services for South Carolina, surveyed 20 middle schools in her state and found to her astonishment that they offered a total of 363 different snack and beverage items for sale—in many cases as alternatives to the regular lunch. The General Accounting Office's 2003 study of the school lunch program reported that 94 percent of high schools and 84 percent of middle schools sell soft drinks or sugary fruit drinks, while about 80 percent of high schools and 60 percent of middle schools sell high-fat cookies, crackers, and salty snacks. Still, students often do have healthier alternatives: 90 percent of high schools also sell fruits and vegetables, and about half offer low-fat yogurt and low-fat cookies or pastries, according to another national study.

In Georgia's Fayette County during 2003, the high school cafeteria's a la carte line regularly sold 144 pounds of French fries each day—

amounting to 5 pounds of French fries per month for every student who bought food in the line! Defending the county school system's decision to offer French fries and other high-fat a la carte items, school nutrition director Cheryl Calhoun told a reporter, "It wasn't something I relished doing, but we had to for our financial survival, plain and simple."

Vending machines have become a seductive source of revenue for school districts. Machines dispensing soft drinks and fruit drinks are featured in the majority of U.S. schools—58 percent of elementary schools, 84 percent of middle schools, and 94 percent of high schools—and school vending machines are often stocked with cookies, candy, and salty snacks as well. Beginning in the early 1990s, soft drink manufacturers looking to expand sales began negotiating exclusivity agreements, known as pouring rights contracts, with many school districts. Under such contracts a district receives substantial payments in exchange for agreeing to stock school vending machines exclusively with a company's products. About 10 percent of the nation's school districts currently have such exclusivity contracts, according to the American Beverage Association (formerly the National Soft Drink Association). One Florida county school board agreed in 2000 to a five-year agreement with Pepsi-Cola worth $13.5 million.

Because so many schools now rely on a la carte and vending machine sales to pay operating costs and fund popular programs, obesity researchers have investigated whether substituting healthier foods and drinks would improve students' diets while still allowing schools to hang on to these lucrative sources of revenue. The answer appears to be yes, if the price of the alternative food items is right. University of Minnesota researcher Simone A. French found that when prices for fresh fruit and baby carrots in a high school cafeteria were cut in half, sales of those items increased twofold to fourfold. In a similar study on high school vending machines, French and her research team found that if the prices of low-fat snacks were set at 50 percent below those of high-fat snacks, sales of the low-fat items doubled. Since total sales from each machine increased, the revenue from vending machines and the profits schools received were unaffected.

The sale of sodas and sugary juice drinks (often containing less

Schools That Allow Food Promotion or Advertising

	Total Schools (%)

Soft Drink Contracts

Schools that have contracts to sell soft drinks:

Elementary schools:	38.2
Middle/junior high:	50.4
Senior high schools:	71.9

Of schools with soft drink contracts, those that:

Receive a specific percentage of soft drink sale receipts	91.7

Receive sales incentives*		
	Elementary schools:	24.0
	Middle/junior high:	40.9
	Senior high schools:	56.7

Allow company advertising in the school building	37.6
Allow company advertising on school grounds	27.7
Allow company advertising on school buses	2.2

Promotion of Candy, Meals from Fast Food Restaurants, and Soft Drinks

Schools that:

Allow promotion through coupons	23.3
Allow promotion through sponsorship of school events	14.3
Allow promotion through school publications	7.7
Prohibit or discourage faculty and staff from using items as rewards	24.8

*Schools receive incentives from companies such as cash awards or donations of equipment or supplies once receipts reach specified amounts. Source: See Notes.

than 10 percent fruit juice) in school vending machines especially worries nutrition experts. Carbonated soft drinks have little or no nutritional value and are the biggest source of added sugars in the diet of American adolescents. In the past two decades soda consumption has doubled among children between the ages of 11 and 17. Kids' daily intake of carbonated drink consumption rises sharply at around the age of 8, and by the time they are 13, U.S. children are drinking more carbonated soft drinks than milk, fruit juice, or fruit drinks. Two-thirds of American adolescent girls and three-quarters of adolescent boys drink soft drinks daily. Evidence indicates that this habit boosts children's total daily calorie intake, apparently because the calories ingested in sodas and other sweetened beverages do not suppress appetite and reduce intake from other sources. In a study of Massachusetts schoolchildren, researchers found that the more sugar-sweetened drinks or soda kids drink each day, the greater their risk of becoming obese.

Armed with research findings like these, parents, pediatricians, nutrition experts, and community activists in many regions have been working to get schools to change their policies regarding what foods and beverages they sell. Measures regulating the foods and drinks that may be sold in school vending machines have been passed or are under consideration in cities and states around the nation. The country's two largest school districts, New York City and Los Angeles, were among the first to act. Soda, candy, salty chips, and sweet snacks like cookies and doughnuts were banned from vending machines in New York City schools starting in September 2003. School authorities also issued new guidelines that reduced the amount of fat allowed in school lunches, prompting cafeterias to come up with low-fat recipes for cheese pizza, chicken fingers, and other entrees. In Los Angeles sodas were banned from vending machines during school hours beginning in January 2004, with a ban on sales of candy, fried chips, and other junk food taking effect later that year. Instead of sodas, school vending machines may dispense water, milk, sports drinks, and fruit-based drinks that contain at least 50 percent juice and no added sweeteners. Student response to the change in Los Angeles was mixed, with some schools reporting a drop in revenues from vending machines when sodas disappeared and others noting brisk sales of the alternative beverages.

In Philadelphia the political mood regarding soda sales in schools shifted radically within a period of less than six months. In August 2003 school district officials were considering an exclusivity contract with a soft drink company that offered $18 million in revenue over a 10-year period. By the following January, after widespread public criticism of the deal, they had retreated from the contract idea and had instead proposed a districtwide ban on school sales of soda and other sweetened beverages.

California has led the way at the state level. A 2001 law sought to ban the sale of soda, candy, and other energy-dense snacks during the school day in elementary schools and to limit soda sales in middle schools, but state budgetary constraints have so far prevented its implementation. Under a separate statewide soda ban enacted in 2003 and taking effect in July 2004, elementary schools can sell only water, milk, and drinks that arc at least 50 percent fruit juice and have no added sweeteners. At middle and junior high schools, sodas may not be sold during regular school hours. Scientists are currently studying the soda ban's impact on obesity rates in California schools.

Texas also recently issued a sweeping new statewide policy on school food, scheduled to be phased in over a five-year period. Under the new rules fried foods would be eliminated from school menus: even French "fries" would have to be baked. Food and drink portions would be downsized and second helpings would be prohibited. In addition, schools would no longer be permitted to sell foods that compete with the cafeteria's official breakfast, lunch, and after-school snack offerings.

The soft drink industry and some school organizations have opposed laws regulating school vending machines, arguing that decisions about what to sell should be left up to local school officials and parents. The industry also contends that efforts to fight obesity should focus on providing kids with more opportunities for physical activity. "It's about the couch, not the can," reads an official statement from the American Beverage Association. "Policymakers should try to increase the quantity and quality of physical education, rather than isolating any one product as the cause of childhood obesity, which soft drinks clearly are not."

But in a sign of the industry's awareness of rising public concern about sodas in schools, the Coca-Cola Company recently revised its guidelines for school partnerships, promising that "carbonated soft drinks will not be made available to students in elementary schools during the school day" and that "a full array of juices, water, and other products will be made available wherever carbonated soft drinks are sold." (Included in the "full array" to be offered to middle school and high school students will be Swerve, Coca-Cola's new milk-based product.) The company also announced that it would no longer offer schools the large one-time payments that had been such a tempting feature of the exclusivity contracts for many districts.

Some critics favor laws that would give the federal government the authority to regulate all foods and drinks sold on school campuses as well as expanded authority to regulate advertising of foods and beverages to children. "The odds are stacked against children and parents when it comes to school vending," nutrition activist Margo Wootan of the nonprofit Center for Science in the Public Interest told a Senate subcommittee in March 2004. "When a parent sends their child to school with lunch money, they do not know if the child will buy a balanced school lunch or a candy bar and a Coke." The expert panel that issued the 2005 IOM report *Preventing Childhood Obesity: Health in the Balance* agrees with that position, urging that all foods and beverages sold or served in schools should be required to meet government nutrition standards. It recommends that the USDA, with advice from an external scientific body, develop new regulations that would specify age-appropriate portion sizes, as well as limit such things as fat and sugar content, in order to establish consistent standards and provide a more healthful food environment for students.

While this policy debate is being played out at the national level, parents can be effective advocates for children locally by monitoring school lunch menus and urging the food service staff to provide healthy meals. They can find out what snacks and beverages are sold in the school store and vending machines. At PTA meetings, parents should raise the issue of foods and drinks sold at school. Some schools have established nutrition committees, composed of representatives from the faculty, administration, student body, food service staff, and parents, to work on improving school fare. In approaching schools, parents would be wise to work with nutrition experts or dietitians in their communities, suggests Leslie A. Lytle, a professor of epidemiology at the University of Minnesota School of Public Health who has done extensive research on obesity prevention programs in schools. "I had a principal say, 'Leslie, you're going to be so happy! The Coke person came around for the vending machines, and I'm asking that they give us Gatorade instead,'" Lytle recalls. Replacing sodas with sweetened sports drinks or with flavored milk products in 16-ounce bottles will not necessarily reduce children's excess calorie intake or help to prevent obesity. Snacks and drinks in schools should not be super-sized, since a package or bottle that contains two or three "portions" is likely to be consumed at one sitting. In deciding what foods and drinks should be available, consider the number of calories an item delivers as well as its content of sugar, fat, saturated fat, trans fats, salt, and nutritionally valuable components such as vitamins and minerals. In all schools, drinking water should be abundantly available, and students should be encouraged to drink water rather than sweetened beverages when thirsty.

🐞🐞🐞

Christine Holmes is a tall, powerfully built woman of color who moves like a dancer. Striding up and down her large open classroom, shaking back her long, curly black hair, she calls out questions to the 20 spellbound seventh-grade students in her health class.

"Dauncy, how many calories equals a pound of fat?"

"Three thousand five hundred," Dauncy says, promptly.

"Raise your hand if you eat just chips for lunch."

Seven or eight hands slowly rise into the air. "Chips and juice," says one boy defensively.

"How many grams of fat in that *small* French fries?"

Fourteen, someone ventures—a guess that's probably a little on the high side.

"How many hours of TV did you watch on Saturday?"

"Seven," admits Cherisse.

"What did you do for the rest?"

"Go out. Hang out with my friends and sister."

Holmes asks how many people have brought in wrappers from their favorite snack foods. One student hands her the wrapping from a cookie bar. She reminds the others to bring in their snack wrappers the following day. "We're going to figure out all the calories in a serving." Then she moves on to discussing last night's homework. "So, why exercise? I asked you to write a little something. Get it out." Eagerly, the students volunteer to read aloud from their essays:

"You could have fun and you can forget about all of your worries."

"To be more athletic."

"To be less embarrassed to be in public."

A shy girl softly reads an entire paragraph about self-confidence. Another girl mentions that exercise keeps your heart healthy. A boy says, "To be strong and to fit in your clothes." Holmes gives everyone a chance to contribute before winding up the discussion: "Americans are overweight. We can stop this, but the only way it can happen is if we exercise."

It's a seamless transition to the next part of the class, a step aerobics session. Holmes asks the students to get up and move their backpacks out of the way. Each boy and girl positions a plastic step platform. Holmes turns on her boom box and puts on a CD of hip-hop music. She starts the students dancing, then marching in place. Soon they're stepping on and off their platforms, moving left and right, punching the air.

"Five, six, seven, eight!" shouts Holmes, moving through the dance steps at the front of the room. "Singles! Doubles! Clap! High up!"

A lot of the kids are grinning now. They pump their arms in time to the music, lifting their knees higher in response to Holmes's exhortations. Three girls are noticeably overweight. They look hot and winded, but like everyone else they keep going. Holmes teaches a dance sequence, then runs the students through the entire routine again. By now they've been doing aerobics for 25 minutes.

At last Holmes leads a slower set of cool-down exercises. "Come on! Don't stop. Don't stop." After a few more minutes she asks them to sit on their platforms and find their pulses. The kids collapse onto the plastic benches, breathing hard and feeling for the artery on the side of the neck. Holmes turns off most of the lights and asks the students to put their heads down and relax quietly for a minute or two. "Today was the first time we did the step routine," she confides to a visitor. "They didn't do too bad at all. I started them with kickboxing first, to invite them into movement. Anything that can get them moving, I'm for it."

Trained to teach health and P.E., Christine Holmes serves as Mildred Avenue Middle School's team leader for Planet Health, an obesity prevention curriculum for students in sixth through eighth grades that is being introduced in many schools in Boston and elsewhere. Mildred Avenue is a newly built middle school adjoining a community center in Mattapan, a low-income neighborhood southwest of downtown Boston. Designed by researchers and educators at the Harvard School of Public Health, Planet Health (mentioned in Chapter 5) integrates lessons on nutrition, physical activity, and reduction of TV time into school curricula in math, language arts, social studies, science, and physical education. It was studied during the late 1990s in a randomized trial involving 10 Boston-area schools, where it reduced children's television viewing, increased fruit and vegetable consumption among girls, and reduced the prevalence of obesity among girls. (Among boys, obesity rates declined in both intervention and control schools; there was no significant difference found between those that received Planet Health and those that did not.) The city's school system has received funding from the federal and state governments and from Blue Cross and Blue Shield of Massachusetts to expand Planet Health, as well as Eat Well & Keep Moving, an elementary school curriculum based on similar principles, into several dozen schools in the Boston area and elsewhere in the state.

Proving that any school curriculum can actually reduce obesity rates has been a difficult task; Planet Health is one of the few to have shown a measurable impact. Harvard's Steven Gortmaker, who led the team that designed it, believes that its effectiveness stems from its simplicity. Planet Health's goal is to impart four basic messages: Be physically active every day. Watch no more than two hours of TV per day. Eat 5 servings of fruits and vegetables every day. Eat fat in moderation.

A research trial is a blunt instrument: it cannot detect all of the effects of changing an educational program. When a school's faculty and staff enthusiastically adopt the principles of a program like Planet Health, there is a more subtle ripple effect on the school community that does not show up in scientific measurements. It manifests itself in unexpected ways. Teachers stop ordering Chinese food for lunch, instead bringing fruit and taking power walks. The guidance counselor drops in to join the aerobics session in Holmes's classroom. The culture of the school starts to change.

This has happened at Mildred Avenue Middle School. Shirley Allen, the principal, moved from a job as principal of another Boston middle school to assume command of the newly built school in September 2003. She brought with her Holmes and several other teachers who had been teaching Planet Health for a year and had been sensitized to the growing concerns about the nutritional value of the foods sold in school cafeterias and vending machines. "For 30 years in this system, I've always had an issue with the food," says Allen, a soft-spoken but forceful woman. "It's kind of odd for me to see a school food system selling foods like potato chips and snacks. A lot of children eat the junk and won't eat the lunch. . . . I have an issue with somebody making money off kids anyway."

A few days before school opened in September, Allen walked into her sparkling new middle school and found a vending machine full of snacks installed in the cafeteria. Outraged, she called a food services official in Boston's school system to protest. A nutritionist assured her that some of the snacks in the machine were healthy. "To me it was so ludicrous," Allen recalls. "I said, 'I don't want it. . . . Take the machine out.'" The next day the snacks had been removed; a week later workmen wheeled away the machine.

This victory emboldened Allen to make other changes. She asked her cafeteria manager to stop selling potato chips and to offer more fresh fruit. She serves water now instead of ginger ale or cider at school council meetings. She has Holmes collaborate with dance and P.E. teachers to put on a quarterly "Fitness Friday" event, an entire day of dance, aerobics, kickboxing, swimming, and other physical activities in which students and many teachers participate. At meetings with other Boston-area principals, she told her colleagues about her success in getting rid of the vending machine. "In the school as a whole, we are more aware [of nutrition]," Allen says. "When there's food in the building for adults, normally you would have a lot of sodas, but pretty much now you just see plain water."

Teachers and administrators at some other Boston-area schools using the new curricula report a similar cultural shift. At Channing Elementary in Hyde Park, another low-income Boston neighborhood, most teachers have received training in the Eat Well & Keep Moving curriculum. Besides lessons in nutrition, they are incorporating aerobics, jump rope, nature walks, and other exercise into their teaching. Classroom-based physical activity is especially important for children at Channing because the century-old school building has no gym or cafeteria, and there is no physical education program. The only place to play is a small paved playground that doubles as a parking area. Principal Deborah Dancy has obtained federal and state funding for a free "healthy breakfast" program at the school and has recruited parents to take turns sending in carrots and celery sticks as snacks for their children's grades. The school nurse compiles a regular newsletter for parents with nutrition tips.

Obesity, diabetes, and high blood pressure are common problems in Hyde Park, including among faculty and staff at Channing. "Quite a few of our teachers have started eating more nutritiously, and they are losing weight," says Dancy. "They have more energy." Equally important, from the principal's viewpoint, are the gains Channing students posted during the 2003–2004 academic year on citywide standardized tests. Dancy says Channing showed the greatest improvement of any school in its local cluster in students' average scores for math and language arts. She credits the Eat Well & Keep Moving curriculum with building her students' mental endurance. "It's not enough just to have the skills," she says. "They have to have the stamina to get through the test."

🐾🐾🐾

Even the best designed and most lavishly funded school programs cannot, by themselves, vanquish the obesity epidemic or ensure that children will be healthy. After years of trying, Leslie Lytle has learned this. The University of Minnesota epidemiologist was a member of the research team that led the CATCH study mentioned in Chapter 5. Conducted among third- through fifth-graders at 96 schools in four states, the three-year trial represented the most exhaustive school-based effort ever undertaken to improve children's habits regarding diet and physical activity. Reducing obesity was not the primary goal of CATCH; its purpose was to improve children's risk profile for heart disease, particularly their blood cholesterol level. However, the project's outcome measures also included children's BMI, body fat, blood pressure, health knowledge, and eating and activity patterns.

CATCH featured a classroom-based health curriculum that taught children about healthy eating, physical activity, and tobacco use. It had a state-of-the-art physical education program designed to increase the time kids spent doing moderate or vigorous activity. And it revamped the school menu to reduce the fat content of lunch offerings. Fifty-six elementary schools were randomly assigned to receive the CATCH intervention; 40 schools served as the control group for comparison.

CATCH succeeded in changing both children's knowledge and their behavior. Children in the intervention schools demonstrated a lasting increase in their knowledge about healthy food choices, and their eating habits actually improved. Compared with students in control schools, CATCH participants lowered their average daily fat intake and spent more time each day being physically active. But these favorable changes were not reflected in the health measurements that determined the trial's scientific outcome. Children in the CATCH program did not show a significant drop in cholesterol or blood pressure, nor did they have lower obesity rates than children in the control schools when the project ended.

Why didn't CATCH reduce children's risk of being overweight? The answer isn't known. Lytle suggests it is still possible that the program did lower the risk, but not soon enough to be apparent when its effects were assessed. Perhaps the benefits will appear later in the participants' lives. Researchers recontacted CATCH participants in the eighth grade, several years after the trial ended, and found that they were still reporting lower fat intake and more physical activity than children in the control group. "They had learned something and it had stuck with them," states Lytle. She is currently restudying CATCH students who are now in twelfth grade, including measuring their BMIs.

CATCH's failure to make a measurable impact on obesity risk may also reflect aspects of the curriculum design. For example, it did not try to persuade children to cut back on how much time they spent watching television, a strategy that has since proved effective in Planet Health and some other school interventions. And although it taught students about healthy food choices, it did not teach them about calories or portion sizes. Obesity prevention researchers are increasingly convinced that those topics need to be included in nutrition education for kids. "Eating a more healthful diet does not necessarily mean you're going to change the energy balance between energy intake and energy output," Lytle notes. "There's the assumption that you'll be eating fewer calories, and that if you're more physically active, you will end up with a weight reduction. I think that's faulty. If we want to study what gets kids to lose weight, we need to design studies that will focus on the energy balance piece of it."

CATCH was school centered. It did not include a major effort to involve families or to change what children did after school or at home. "While we could positively affect the school piece, kids' total calorie intake and energy expenditure is over a 24-hour period," Lytle points out. "The family is a huge piece of this. We're really struggling about how to get families engaged in all health promotions with kids." CATCH was also an enormous project: it included more than 5,000 children in different regions of the country. How effectively the program was implemented varied, Lytle says, depending on the leadership and enthusiasm at individual schools. The same would undoubtedly be true of any new program a school system adopted.

After years of doing research in schools, "I can walk into a new school and almost within an hour say, 'This school, if there's a randomized intervention, will be dynamite,' or 'This school will be hard,'" Lytle states. "You can feel it. . . . Schools where there's more cohesion, felt support, and all those kinds of things tend to adopt and institutionalize health programs much more aggressively than schools that are disconnected and struggling." Leadership, a sense of purpose, clear educational principles, passionate and energetic teachers, adequate space and resources, involvement by parents and by the local community—the same qualities a school needs to effectively teach reading and math are what it needs to teach children how to be healthy.

Sometimes the best way to find an educational strategy that works is to start small. In 2001, when Meg Campbell started Codman Academy, a tiny public charter school in Boston's Dorchester neighborhood, she drew on all the lessons she had learned as a teacher, poet, community organizer, health care researcher, mother of two daughters, and former "chubby kid." Campbell believes that a central flaw in American education is that schools concentrate on nurturing children's minds but fail to nurture their bodies. She had helped start Expeditionary Learning Outward Bound, a school reform project focused on active learning, and had been following the research findings on childhood obesity and physical activity. When she was planning her charter school, Campbell says, she was "immersed in the healthy mind/healthy body connection." She decided she wanted to found a school where walking was built into the daily routine. She took a map of Dorchester, placed the point of her compass on the new school's headquarters (located in the community health center at Codman Square), and drew a circle with a 1-mile radius. "I figured a mile was about the most that kids would walk" at one time, she says. She arranged her students' schedule so that they had to walk to classes and activities scattered around the neighborhood, up to a mile apart: a tennis center, a gym, various classroom settings.

In its third year of operation, Codman Academy is a tough college preparatory school with approximately 80 students in grades 9 through 11. Most are African American children from poor families. They walk an average of 6 miles per week in addition to attending regular physical education classes (including required tennis). "If you do not like walking, this might not be the right school for you," wrote ninth-grader Marquis Benjamin in a letter to new students. "When I first came here, I did not like to walk a lot but then one of my teachers said that I would have to learn to like it. . . . Now it does not really bother me as much." Walking has become part of the school culture. Campbell tells her students that, just like Codman's strict academic standards, the walking is preparing them for higher education: "It's like college. In college, you walk everywhere."

"I have some kids who are really clinically obese," she says. "They'll break into a sweat walking." Many of the school's approximately 80 students have lost weight since they enrolled at Codman, including one girl who has lost 50 pounds. "No one has gained weight at our school," Campbell says proudly. She puts nutrition lessons in the curriculum, puts scales in the bathrooms, and makes sure lunch offerings are healthy. In contracts with food vendors she specifies that she will accept no French fries, no sausage, no high-fat items. "Many people in education say, 'I have no control over lunch.' They say, 'Kids don't like lettuce.' I say, 'Well, they don't usually walk in saying, 'Please, can I have algebra?' either."

Codman students attend classes from 9 a.m. to 5 p.m. Mondays through Fridays and from 9 a.m. to noon on Saturdays. Campbell can't prevent her teenage students from going to the McDonald's across the street and buying lunch or snacks, but she forbids them to bring the food onto school premises. She tells them, "You know how I feel about it. It's like cigarettes. If you want to clog your arteries, do it on your own time." She doesn't buy the argument that fighting obesity is outside the realm of public schools' responsibility. She believes that children want to be healthy, want to eat right, and feel empowered by knowing how to take care of their bodies.

"We have an epidemic, and the biggest contributor to the epidemic as far as I can see is public schools—both in terms of the poor food that they give and the lack of exercise," she says. "It's nothing to do with personal choice, because the kids are captive, at least for nine months of the year. This is a public health problem that we can solve."

CHAPTER 8

Finding Help for an Overweight Child

Trianna is sending out signals of distress. At each of her past appointments with dietitian Erika Zeff, the 13-year-old girl has been cheerful, voluble, and enthusiastic. But at tonight's meeting in an examining room at the University of Virginia's "fitness clinic," she sits silently beside her mother, her big dark eyes focused on the floor. When Zeff asks Trianna a question, the teenager often looks at her mom, waiting for her to answer first. Then, more often than not, she takes issue with the answer.

The fitness clinic was established at the University of Virginia Medical Center to teach overweight Charlottesville youngsters and their families how to make changes in diet, activity, and lifestyle. Thanks to a research grant, treatment is free. Zeff is a registered dietitian, but during her monthly appointments with Trianna she also plays the roles of psychologist, nurse, cheerleader, and personal trainer, drawing on her people skills and her intuition about what makes families tick. The clinic's medical treatment plan is designed and supervised by Milagros Huerta, a pediatrician trained in endocrinology and obesity treatment; a psychologist provides training and backup for staff in behavior modification techniques. Zeff is the person who sees the majority of the clinic's young patients at their monthly visits. It's her first real job after completing her internship as a clinical dietitian, and she looks almost as young as some of the teenagers she is treating. Warm, energetic, and confident, she seems well suited to coaching kids in the difficult task of changing their eating habits.

Trianna has been coming to the clinic for several months. Dressed in a bright red polo shirt and shorts, the young African American girl looks fairly fit but carries some extra weight around her middle. Since enrolling in the program she had been losing weight steadily, but tonight, for the first time, her weight is up slightly. Zeff suspects she's getting tired of following the regimen. She runs through the list of goals Trianna set for herself at their last meeting. Is she eating breakfast every day? Yes, Trianna says. But her breakfast—a juice drink and a package of peanut butter crackers—usually is consumed during a midmorning break in classes, more than three hours after she boards the school bus each morning.

Is she measuring her serving sizes?

"No, not really," Trianna admits. "But I don't eat chips anymore."

How has she been doing on her activity goals?

Her pedometer count is up to about 5,000 steps a day, Trianna reports. She has been practicing with a dance team five days a week and goes to a "steps" exercise workout on Saturdays. She plays basketball for an hour one or two afternoons each week at a local youth club. Zeff is impressed by the amount of physical activity she is doing.

"When are you hungriest?" Zeff asks.

When she comes home from school, Trianna replies. Her mother is still at work then, she adds, and "I can't find anything to eat."

"So what do you actually eat?"

"Oodles of Noodles," admits Trianna. "Half a container."

"That's OK," Zeff tells her. "It's not the healthiest, but at least you're only eating half."

Trianna's mother says she is worried that the fat on Trianna's abdomen is not coming off fast enough. She's afraid her daughter will become the target of teasing. "She is going to high school in September," she says. "High school kids, they're mean."

Zeff reminds her that changing unhealthy habits is more important than losing pounds rapidly. She turns to Trianna. "Are you maybe getting a little tired of all this?" she asks. "Is it hard for you?" Trianna says no. This time her mother is the one who jumps in to contest the answer.

"You were telling me it was hard," she reminds her daughter. "We were in the kitchen and I was fixing something, sweet potato pie." Trianna's sister—the "skinny one" in the family—was expected home from college. "You said, 'That's not fair that I can't have it!' You always say it's hard. I think I did give you just a little slice."

Zeff smiles sympathetically. She asks Trianna whether she has been getting regular nonfood rewards for sticking with her eating and activity guidelines. She turns to the sheet of paper where she has been listing Trianna's goals for the coming month. She helps Trianna and her mother negotiate an agreement about an activity they can do together: Trianna's mother likes to go for walks in a large cemetery near their house, but Trianna would rather have her mom take bike rides with her. "I'll put down that if you do five days of your goals, nutrition, and exercise, you get something special," Zeff says. "Maybe a privilege."

Trianna grins. "Stay out late!" she crows.

For the parents of an overweight child, locating high-quality treatment—and figuring out how to pay for it—can be challenging. Although just about everyone agrees that the steeply rising rates of obesity in American children and adults constitute an epidemic, obesity itself is not yet fully recognized as a disease. In most cases, weight-loss treatment for an overweight child or adult is not covered by health insurance unless and until the excess body fat produces a complication that is universally recognized as a disease. The commonest such complications in overweight kids include diabetes or high insulin levels, high blood pressure, and high blood levels of cholesterol or triglycerides. However, obese children are also at risk for developing a variety of other medical problems.

Fortunately, rising national concern about the health impact of the obesity epidemic is gradually beginning to prompt changes in the position of health insurers. In 2004 policymakers at the U.S. Department of Health and Human Services declared that obesity would no longer be automatically excluded from the list of conditions whose treatments were eligible for coverage by the federal government's vast Medicare program. They instructed Medicare officials to begin collecting data to determine which types of weight-loss treatment were effective and should be paid for. Although Medicare primarily covers the elderly, its policy decisions influence those of other insurers. Specialists in pediatric obesity treatment note that a few other health insurance programs have covered such treatment for children in selected cases; more will likely begin to do so in the future.

Helping overweight children achieve a healthier weight as early as possible—*before* they develop medical complications from the excess weight—is clearly the best way to improve their long-term health outlook. Yet the incentives currently built into the medical insurance system seem designed to discourage prevention and prompt, early treatment not just for obesity but for many other diseases. This has created a situation in which surgery for severe obesity—most commonly a major abdominal operation that is highly effective at producing weight loss but has the potential for life-threatening complications—is covered by insurance and is being performed on very obese teenagers with weight-related medical conditions at some U.S. hospitals. Meanwhile, nutritional counseling and behavioral treatment for less severely overweight children and their families aimed at improving eating and activity habits—although safe and in many cases effective—is usually not covered by insurance and as a result is difficult for many families to obtain.

In the past doctors sometimes advised parents of an overweight child not to worry about the excess weight, reassuring them that their child would probably "grow out of" being fat during the growth spurt that occurs before puberty in girls and during early adolescence in boys. That advice may still hold true for some moderately overweight kids, but in general today's pediatricians are being urged to be more proactive in trying to change the eating and activity habits of overweight children and their families. In part, this is because American kids are heavier now than ever before, making it unlikely that many of today's overweight boys and girls will "grow into" their weight as they mature. Current American Academy of Pediatrics guidelines recommend that all children whose BMIs are at or above the 95th percentile for their age—as well as children with BMIs between the 85th and 95th percentiles who have any medical condition associated with obesity—should be evaluated and considered for treatment.

What we know about the biology of children's bodies favors early treatment. Evidence suggests that treating overweight kids before they go through puberty may be more likely to produce substantial and sustained weight loss than waiting until a fat child has become a fat adolescent. Some of the hormonal and physiological changes associated with puberty, particularly in girls, tend to facilitate weight gain and to make weight loss more difficult. Puberty in both sexes may also be associated with changes in brain centers that regulate appetite and body weight, tending to "lock in" a particular level of fat stores as the body's set point. Adolescents, especially girls, are less physically active on average than younger kids.

For girls, being overweight can make puberty begin earlier and can lead to specific hormonal changes related to the reproductive system, fertility, and possibly future breast cancer risk. High body weight is associated with an earlier age of first menstruation, apparently because hormonal signals from body fat stores influence the age at which a girl enters puberty. In turn, girls who start menstruating at a young age have a higher lifetime risk of breast cancer than those who start later. Obesity in adolescent girls is also a risk factor for a disorder of the ovaries that can cause menstrual irregularities and infertility. "Puberty is a risk factor [for excess weight gain] for girls more than it is for boys," notes Leonard Epstein, a nationally known expert in treating overweight children. Women's bodies have evolved to prepare for childbearing: with the onset of puberty, the female sex hormones estrogen and progesterone tend to promote the deposition of fat as an energy depot that the body can use to sustain a future pregnancy. In addition, perhaps as a behavioral response to hormonal factors, girls entering puberty tend to reduce their level of physical activity.

As children approach the teenage years, their increasing desire for independence may also make them more reluctant to cooperate with family-based treatment aimed at changing their eating and activity habits. Parents usually have more influence on the behavior of their kids during the preschool and elementary school years than they do once their offspring are adolescents. The dietary habits of kids during elementary school are also less firmly established and easier for parents to change than are the eating habits of older children, and the food environment and opportunities for physical activity are usually better in elementary schools than in middle schools and high schools.

Perhaps as a result of a combination of biological, social, and environmental factors, preadolescent kids aged 6 or older who are obese have about a 50-50 chance of still being obese when they grow up, while obese teenagers have about a 75 percent chance of becoming obese adults. (In children younger than 3 years old, being fat has been found not to predict future obesity risk.)

The best-documented and most lasting success in treating obese children has been achieved by specialized multidisciplinary teams of professionals who work with the entire family to change eating and physical activity habits. Epstein's program, which he started in Pittsburgh and has continued in Buffalo, has the longest track record with this approach. In 1994 Epstein reported the results of 10 years of follow-up among 158 children he had treated for obesity. All of the kids had been between the ages of 8 and 12 when they and their families participated in his program, whose primary strategy was reducing children's calorie intake and promoting healthier eating habits by a combination of a diet, modifying the home environment, and teaching parents to use behavior modification techniques to reward positive changes. Ten years after being treated, 30 percent of the children were not obese. In a subset of children whose treatment had combined diet with "lifestyle exercise" (allowing the kids to choose the kinds and amount of physical activity they did and rewarding them for doing it), the success rate was higher: a decade after treatment, 50 percent were not obese. These figures compare favorably with the results achieved by most weight-loss treatment programs for obese adults. Many studies have found that within five years after losing weight by following treatment programs, 90 to 95 percent of overweight adults have regained the pounds they had lost.

A number of behavioral treatment programs, including the University of Virginia's fitness clinic in Charlottesville, have been based wholly or partly on Leonard Epstein's model. Many use an eating plan based on his Stoplight Diet, which I describe in more detail later in this chapter. Some other experts note that the families in Epstein's program were very highly motivated and say that the success rate in achieving long-term weight loss among children who went through his intensive program has been difficult to match in other communities. "Successful behavioral programs are labor intensive, are not yet translated into versions that can easily be applied on the primary care level, and require intensive parental involvement which, for many families, is simply not realistic," write NIH obesity researchers Jack and Susan Yanovski in a recent assessment of the current state of treatment for overweight children.

Epstein acknowledges that achieving comparable long-term success rates with his obesity treatment program today may be more difficult than it was when he started in the 1980s. The children entering his program today are twice as obese, on average, as the those he treated 20 years ago. That shift reflects the fact that, in addition to the recent increase in the number of overweight kids in the United States, the proportion who are severely obese has grown. He and his team have found that once children have become very obese—weighing twice as much, or more, than they should weigh for their height—it becomes more difficult for them to lose weight.

Assembling a multidisciplinary team to treat obese children is expensive for a hospital or clinic. Typically, it includes a pediatrician (often an endocrinologist, a specialist in hormone disorders), a clinical dietitian, one or more nurses or nurse practitioners, a psychologist trained in behavioral treatment, and sometimes a social worker and an exercise physiologist skilled in developing and monitoring physical activity programs for kids. Since insurance in most cases will not pay for such services, few medical centers have been able to make the investment, even though treatment for overweight kids is urgently needed all over the United States. Even in those cities that do have state-of-the-art behavioral treatment programs for obese children and their families, such programs are often supported almost entirely by government research grants; children sometimes must be enrolled in clinical research studies in order to be treated.

Parents can find federally funded research programs on childhood obesity by searching a Web site maintained by the National Institutes of Health. (See page 271 in Resources.) NIH officials caution that the research institutes cannot recommend individual treatment programs since they have no way to assess or monitor the quality of clinical care provided.

"I would say that of all the difficulties parents will face" in finding treatment for an overweight child, "the biggest are, first of all, trying to find people who know how to do it, and also trying to find affordable care," says Robert Berkowitz, a psychiatrist who treats obese adolescents as part of a research program at the University of Pennsylvania in Philadelphia. "It's a paradox: here we are in an epidemic, and yet we have very few programs."

Epstein's findings and those of other pediatric researchers treating obesity have established some general principles about the most effective strategies for getting kids to change their eating habits, reduce their daily calorie intake, and become more active. An important point to remember is that children differ from adults both physically and psychologically. Parents should not unilaterally decide to put their child on a diet or sign a teenager up for the commercial weight-loss program that worked for them. Consulting a child's primary care doctor should always be the first step for parents worried about whether their child needs to lose weight. In making decisions about treatment, the pediatrician or family physician will consider whether the parents are also overweight and whether there is a family history of obesity or of related diseases, such as diabetes, high blood pressure, or heart disease, as well as review the child's overall health and growth records. The physician will also want to talk with the child alone, to find out how the child feels about his or her body and to ask questions that assess mood, eating patterns, and overall mental health.

In addition to outlining the kinds of treatment approaches for overweight kids likely to be available in many communities, I will briefly discuss treatments that are considered experimental or contro-versial in children or teenagers. The latter include prescription weight-loss drugs and bariatric surgery (operations that induce weight loss by reducing stomach capacity and/or changing the anatomy of the diges-tive tract to decrease absorption of food).

🐾🐾🐾

Sometimes it's a mother or father who first becomes worried that a child is becoming overweight; sometimes it's the pediatrician or family doctor. And sometimes it's the child who comes home from school and reports that classmates have begun to tease him or her about being fat. In any case, the first step is for child and parents (or at least one parent) to sit down with the child's doctor to review the growth and health records and to talk about the family's medical history and hab-its. It's important to discuss whether the child is taking any prescrip-tion or over-the-counter medicines or supplements. Certain drugs, including steroids, some antiseizure medicines, and some medications used to treat depression or psychiatric illnesses, can cause considerable weight gain.

By asking questions and performing a physical examination, your doctor can usually determine whether there is any reason to suspect an identifiable medical cause for the excessive weight gain, such as a hor-mone disorder or one of the extremely rare genetic mutations that produce obesity (discussed in Chapter 2). Hormone and genetic disor-ders cause far fewer than 10 percent of cases of childhood obesity and are usually easy for doctors to distinguish from "idiopathic obesity"—obesity of unknown cause—which accounts for the vast majority of cases. Children who are fat because of hormonal or genetic disorders are usually short for their age and have symptoms or physical charac-teristics that provide clues to their diagnosis. Also, their bone growth and development are typically delayed for their age, a feature that can easily be evaluated on an X-ray. In contrast, most children with idio-pathic obesity are taller than average for their age and have no unusual physical characteristics or delayed bone growth. They often enter pu-berty earlier than their peers. Most overweight children do not need to undergo a battery of expensive laboratory tests to seek a medical ex-planation for their weight problem.

On the other hand, certain medical tests *are* recommended for kids whose BMI is at the 85th percentile or higher for their age. These tests are done to screen for common medical problems that can be caused by being overweight, such as high cholesterol or triglycerides in the blood, high blood pressure, and diabetes or a prediabetic condition in which the body's response to glucose is abnormal and insulin levels are high.

Special attention is often required when examining overweight children. They frequently need a specially sized blood pressure cuff to measure pressure accurately. The doctor should also question the child about headaches, hip or knee pain, snoring, and daytime sleepiness and should carefully check eyes and leg joints. (Snoring and sleepiness can be symptoms of sleep apnea, an obesity-related disorder in which breathing becomes obstructed during sleep. The other parts of the examination help screen for potentially serious neurologic and orthopedic complications of being overweight.)

Checking for obesity-associated medical problems helps the doctor and family plan the next steps in treatment. For example, an abnormally high fasting blood glucose level in a child whose BMI is at the 85th percentile would signal the need to test more extensively for a prediabetic condition and would increase the urgency of addressing the child's weight. Identifying any medical condition associated with obesity would also mean that the family's health insurance would be more likely to cover the obesity treatment.

Nancy McLaren, clinical associate professor of pediatrics and medical director of the Teen Health Center at the University of Virginia in Charlottesville, explains that her first priority in talking with parents of an overweight child is to get them to recognize their child's weight as a health problem. Many families are not aware of the potential medical consequences of a child's obesity and may not have been concerned about it. "We talk initially about what the family history is of diabetes or heart problems," she said. "I start from the perspective of trying to make them see that their child is moving into that. You're used to Grandma having [such diseases] at 65 or 70. We even have some patients in their teens now that have these problems."

McLaren assesses her patients' mental health and asks about eating disorders such as binge eating disorder or bulimia nervosa, in which loss of control of eating is followed by vomiting or other purging behaviors. She finds that children's attitudes about their bodies are strongly influenced by standards of beauty within their culture or ethnic group: for example, white girls often want to weigh less, but some African American girls want to weigh more. "I always ask them how they feel about themselves and their bodies," she says. "That's where I get 'I'm too fat' or 'I don't weigh enough.'" Parents and doctors need to find out about such perceptions before they focus on changing a child's eating habits. "You want to be careful with kids, because kids can become obsessed," McLaren cautions. Sometimes, when trying to reduce their food intake, "what you can see is, these kids lose weight and then go to the other extreme." Such a response to treatment is rare, however. Parents should not allow fears about inducing an eating disorder to preclude sensible and healthful attempts to address a child's weight problem.

McLaren next questions the child and parent in detail about eating and activity patterns. "It takes a long time," she says. "I try to look at where most of the calories are coming from. I try to talk about what initial small changes they can make" within that framework. She focuses especially on her young patients' intake of sodas, sugary drinks, and juice; their snacking habits; and their calcium intake. Her goal is to look for obvious ways to help the child or teenager cut back on sugar and fat intake and boost intake of whole grains and of calcium, whether from nonfat dairy products or other sources. A high calcium intake—from dairy foods, other sources rich in this element, or supplements—is recommended for children and teenagers to aid in bone development. Preliminary evidence also suggests that a high calcium intake, particularly from nonfat or low-fat dairy sources, may reduce fat storage by the body and facilitate weight loss. Some nutrition experts are skeptical of these findings, pointing out that some of the research that yielded these results was paid for by the dairy industry. Additional larger and longer-running studies are needed in order to confirm them.

Based on the information she gathers, McLaren usually works with each overweight patient to come up with a simple plan, one containing just a few steps the child and family can take to cut back on high-calorie foods or drinks. For example, "We might talk about cutting back to one soda a day from four," she states. "I tell them, if they are going to drink fruit juice, to use 100 percent juice and to have one 8-ounce glass a day. Then the rest of the time, try to drink only water."

Another effective strategy is to ask patients what "white foods" they are eating. The list might include white bread, white pasta, white potatoes, and white rice. She routinely suggests that they cut back on such foods, switching when possible to darker-colored, whole grain alternatives (or perhaps, in the case of potatoes, choosing sweet potatoes or squash). Whole grains contain more fiber and more vitamins and are also digested more slowly than processed grains, a factor that may help reduce hunger between meals. The 2005 edition of the federal government's dietary guidelines, being prepared as this book goes to press, is expected to urge Americans to try to choose whole grain products such as whole wheat bread or brown rice instead of refined products like white bread or white rice.

McLaren advises her patients to cut back on pasta and other starches, opting sometimes to have a small portion of meat, chicken, or fish and ample portions of vegetables instead of including a starch in every main meal. She talks to them about reading food labels and measuring portion sizes. She sometimes suggests that her teenage patients use an inexpensive food handbook published for users of the South Beach Diet as a pocket-size resource to help them choose foods relatively low in sugar, fat, and refined carbohydrates. (She does not, however, recommend that her teenagers follow the South Beach Diet's "induction" phase, which she considers overly restrictive.)

The Stoplight Diet, an eating plan developed by Leonard Epstein in the 1980s, is another approach to changing children's eating habits that has been widely and successfully used by pediatricians and dietitians. Calling it a diet is something of a misnomer: like David Ludwig's OWL plan (discussed in Chapter 4), the Stoplight approach teaches kids healthy lifelong eating patterns. Rather than forbidding any specific food, it groups foods into "green," "yellow," and "red" categories based on their calorie content by weight (energy density). Most vegetables, except starchy ones like potatoes and beans, have low energy density and are green foods. Candy, cookies, sweet desserts, butter, oils, pizza, and high-fat snacks or fast food items are energy dense and are therefore red foods. The majority of foods, such as fruits, bread and cereal, starchy vegetables, fish, eggs, and meat, fall into the yellow category. They are intermediate in energy density and low or moderate in fat and provide vitamins, minerals, fiber, and complex carbohydrates or protein. Yellow foods are the mainstay of the eating plan but are to be eaten cautiously, with careful attention to portion size. Children are encouraged to eat as much of the green foods as they want. Red foods are to be eaten only occasionally and in small amounts, and parents are urged to banish them from the home if possible.

The principle behind the Stoplight Diet is that low-energy-density foods like vegetables can help satisfy hunger without contributing too many calories to a child's daily intake. By following it, kids learn to eat a low-fat, nutritionally balanced diet that emphasizes lots of vegetables and fruits and to avoid foods high in simple sugars or fat. "If you eat a bigger volume of low-calorie food, you will feel full," Epstein says. He also recommends about 2 servings a day of nonfat dairy products. And kids should be allowed to have their favorite snacks or treats on occasion, even if those items are red foods. In working to change children's and teenagers' eating behavior, McLaren notes, a cardinal rule is not to make strict prohibitions. "Never do an absolute thing," she says. "Never say, 'Don't do this anymore.'"

Incorporating more physical activity into the daily routine should be part of any strategy for helping a child attain a healthier weight. Overweight children have poorer endurance than lean kids and are often reluctant to exercise. Treatment guidelines suggest that overweight kids should initially be physically active for at least 30 minutes a day, the minimum recommended for all children in a report by the U.S. Surgeon General. But more recent recommendations for all children urge a minimum of 60 minutes of moderate to vigorous exercise daily, a goal that overweight kids should work toward achieving. Physical activity will make it easier for kids to stabilize their weight, will help make them fitter, and will increase their chances of keeping off any pounds they lose.

McLaren's approach to physical activity is similar to that for food intake: she starts by questioning her patients about their daily routines, how much TV they watch, and their opportunities for building in exercise. She urges them to cut back on the time they spend watching television or playing computer games. "We talk about walking. Where can you walk to rather than ride to? Are there exercises you can do at home—can you put on music and dance? Could you park farther away at the mall—or walk around more while you're there?" Many of her young patients cannot safely ride bicycles in their neighborhoods, but they may have access to playgrounds or community recreation centers. McLaren urges them to play basketball, go bowling or rollerblading, dance, or play with hula hoops. "The kids who are really obese, I don't want them going out and running," she says.

Leonard Epstein's best results for achieving sustained weight loss have come from combining dietary changes with "lifestyle exercise," in which kids earned points by doing any of a variety of physical activities. Letting the child choose the activity is a key feature of the program's success. "Children could get exercise points as long as they did at least 10 minutes of something," he says. "They could walk back and forth to school. They could play on the playground. It didn't have to be aerobic exercise." Aerobic exercise is better for fitness—it conditions the heart, lungs, and muscles to work more efficiently—but frequent periods of lower-intensity exercise can be very effective in helping people achieve and maintain weight loss. "Weight loss depends on energy expenditure, not the intensity," Epstein states.

Obesity experts emphasize that overweight kids and their families should try to make just a few small permanent changes at a time. Once they have succeeded in incorporating those changes, they can build on them by going on to the next step. Too much information at once or too drastic a revision of a child's and family's lifestyle are likely to be overwhelming and frustrating for everybody. Epstein urges parents to keep in mind that in helping an overweight child the goal is not to instantly transform habits or to drop pounds overnight. That's one of the ways a good treatment plan for children differs from commercial weight-loss programs for adults. "Adult weight control programs get evaluated by how much you lose and how fast you lose," Epstein says. "With kids the speed at which they develop healthy habits is not nearly as important as how permanent they are."

For many children, parents can achieve a lot simply by changing the food environment at home to get rid of calorie-dense snacks, drinks, and sweets, by reducing TV time, and by improving their own eating and exercise habits. It's important for the whole family to make a commitment to a healthier lifestyle. "I bet you lots of kids would benefit tremendously by the parents really moderating the eating and exercise environment and adopting healthier behavior—and not even talking to the kids about changing," Epstein says. "They would just change automatically."

Current guidelines for doctors treating overweight kids advise that in setting up a treatment plan the first step in weight control for all overweight children over 2 years old should be trying to maintain the current weight. Since children are growing in height, a child's BMI will automatically decrease as he or she grows if body weight remains stable. For many children, modest changes in diet and activity will be enough to keep the weight steady. If a child and family can achieve this, they are already succeeding. For some kids, especially those whose BMI is between the 85th and 95th percentiles for age and who do not have medical complications, continuing to maintain a steady weight under a pediatrician's supervision can provide a safe, gradual way to get to a healthier BMI as the child continues to grow.

Children whose BMI is above the 95th percentile, as well as kids who have already achieved most of their growth and those who have medical complications caused by being overweight, are likely to need to make additional changes in diet and activity once their weight has stabilized in order to lose some of the excess fat. They should be monitored regularly by a doctor and, if possible, by a dietitian. Current treatment guidelines suggest that the goal in most cases should be to lose weight at a rate of about 1 to 4 pounds per month. The child and family should work with the doctor to set realistic goals. Although many overweight kids (like many overweight adults) dream of looking like the actors, pop stars, or athletes they see on television, those body types are not possible for everyone. Developing permanent, healthy habits and choosing an achievable BMI goal should be the priorities. "These are habit-changing programs. These are lifelong programs," advises psychiatrist Robert Berkowitz. A pitfall of many adult weight-control programs is that people think of them as a short-term fix, after which they will be able to revert to their old habits. "That model doesn't work," he says. "Right from the beginning, we say to people that this is a lifelong issue."

Severe restrictions on caloric intake in children can interfere with growth, and unsupervised efforts to achieve rapid weight loss can lead to vitamin deficiencies, eating disorders, and other medical problems. Any child who has a serious or life-threatening medical illness requiring rapid weight loss should be treated by a specialist in pediatric obesity. The best way for parents to find such physicians, or to locate high-quality programs specializing in obesity treatment in children, is to call the office of the department of pediatrics at local medical schools or the nearest children's hospital.

What factors have been found to contribute to a positive outcome? Much research on behavior change, including studies of obesity treatments, has shown that long-term success depends on the participants' ability to monitor their own behavior. That doesn't necessarily require counting calories, but a child's treatment plan should include some way of keeping track of the kinds of food and drink, the portion sizes, and the number of servings the child has each day. Similarly, it should include a system for recording the type and duration of exercise, as well as "screen" time: hours spent watching TV, playing video games, or sitting at the computer. Keeping track of daily diet and activity patterns will help motivate the child and family and will make it easier to identify specific factors that might be interfering with success—such as problem foods or situations that trigger impulsive snacking. The parents, the doctor, and the child undergoing treatment should discuss how often the child will be weighed and who will be responsible for weighing and recording weights. Among overweight teenagers treated at the University of Pennsylvania's treatment program, "those kids who actively monitor their food intake and exercise and have pretty good estimates of their calorie consumption—those are the kids who actually do pretty well," says Berkowitz.

Another element common to successful programs is a requirement that the entire family should be on board, as well as caregivers who spent significant amounts of time with the child. Treatment plans tend to fail when they focus only on the overweight child, imposing different rules for that child than for the rest of the family. Programs in which least one parent goes along to each treatment session are also more likely to work, although parents and children often meet in separate groups during the sessions, especially if the program is treating adolescents. In Leonard Epstein's program, parents do more than simply learn the rules: they are given the same diet as their child and are also asked to follow their own exercise program. "I would guess probably two-thirds of the parents are clinically obese, and . . . almost all probably could either improve the quality of their diet or improve their physical activity—so there's plenty to target," he says. "They have to model healthier behaviors. They also see what the kid's going through."

The psychological component of Epstein's program and others like it is probably the most difficult part for parents to learn and the most difficult and costly feature to replicate in community treatment settings, yet the techniques families learn from psychologists and counselors are critical to long-term treatment success. A key technique is contingency contracting, in which parent and child sign a weekly or monthly contract in which the child earns rewards if he or she succeeds in reaching mutually agreed upon short-term goals, such as cutting TV time by an hour a day or switching from drinking soda to drinking water. Rather than food or expensive prizes, rewards should be an activity that the parent and child can do together, like going to a movie or hosting a pajama party. Children and adults can also sign contracts in which a child promises to reward a parent. (For example: "I promise to let you sleep late on Saturday morning if you will play Frisbee with me after dinner two nights this week.")

Other important behavior change techniques for parents include learning to praise children on a daily basis, especially for performing a desired new behavior such as keeping track of portion sizes or recording TV time in a diary; avoiding being critical or making negative comments; acting consistently; restructuring the home environment to contain fewer temptations and more healthy options; and helping the child figure out strategies in advance for dealing with difficult situations such as parties or visits to restaurants.

At a Stanford University treatment program for overweight children between 8 and 12 years old, parents and kids start each weekly session together by weighing in and talking about how the week has gone. They review not just their dietary intake, but how well they did at remembering to praise each other. They examine how many points the kids earned for following the eating plan, reducing TV time, and exercising. Then adults and children meet in separate groups with program staff to discuss their progress during the preceding week in greater detail, to ask questions, and to plan new goals. Parents and children sign new contracts, agreeing on goals and rewards to be earned during the week to come. The program uses an eating plan based on the Stoplight approach. "We don't put kids on diets. We help them eat more healthfully," says Stanford researcher Tom Robinson. "If they are losing more than 1 pound a week, we look to see if they are skipping meals."

Research data collected at Stanford, as well as data from Epstein's studies and other programs, suggest that such an approach helps kids lose weight without promoting obsessive or disordered eating patterns. "We do focus on weight loss—that's what they come to us for," Robinson says. "We know that overweight girls, to start with, are at higher risk of bulimia and, probably, anorexia nervosa. . . . We measure weight concerns in girls. To date, we haven't seen anything get worse— mostly, we see it get better. We believe that by promoting healthful behavior changes, we can reduce the risk for eating disorders."

🐾🐾🐾

Some families will find that several visits with a pediatrician and dietitian, combined with a concerted effort to change their eating and exercise routines, help their overweight child achieve a healthier BMI. However, a severely obese child or one who has suffered a medical complication of obesity needs specialized treatment at the outset. Parents should ask their pediatrician for help in finding the best treatment program in their region. Many other children could probably benefit from something in between.

What about commercial weight-loss programs? Pediatric treatment guidelines do not recommend commercial programs designed for adults, such as Weight Watchers or Jenny Craig, for children because no studies exist of their effectiveness in kids. In a recent assessment of the current state of treatment for overweight kids, NIH researchers Jack and Susan Yanovski cautioned that doctors should not automatically assume that adult weight-loss programs (or other options, such as drugs) will work and be safe in young children.

Still, commercial programs may be a reasonable option for some motivated adolescents who have obtained their doctor's and parents' permission. Parents should thoroughly familiarize themselves with the program's approach, and parents and doctor should carefully consider the boy's or girl's overall health, eating habits, and personality makeup in deciding whether to permit enrollment.

A spokeswoman for Jenny Craig said the program accepts adolescents 13 and older who have no preexisting health conditions as long as a parent provides permission for them to participate. Weight Watchers International revised its policy in 2003 to more strictly limit access to its programs by children and adolescents. Kids between the ages of 10 and 16 may participate only if they have both a parent's signature and a doctor's referral that includes an individualized weight goal or range.

A few commercial programs have been developed specifically for children, but little scientific research has been done to evaluate their long-term effectiveness. The Shapedown Pediatric Obesity Program, developed in the 1980s by researchers at the University of California, San Francisco, is a commercially licensed program for children, teenagers, and their parents. An older program, it is offered in many U.S. cities and has probably been used by thousands of families. The only published scientific trial of its effectiveness was done in adolescents between the ages of 12 and 18. The 1987 study compared 37 overweight kids who were randomly assigned to receive the 14-session program combining dietary change, exercise, and behavioral counseling, with 29 kids receiving no treatment. Children in the treatment group lost weight (an average of about 7 pounds) during the three-month program, while those in the control group did not. The study suggested that Shapedown participants derived some benefit for at least a year. No studies providing longer follow-up or more recent results for Shapedown participants have been published.

Committed to Kids is a treatment program for obese adolescents developed at Louisiana State University's Pennington Biomedical Research Center in Baton Rouge. The program is promoted in the book *Trim Kids* by LSU exercise physiologist Melinda S. Sothern and two colleagues. The Committed to Kids curriculum, patient materials, and training manuals are marketed to health professionals on a Web site, so some families may find the program in their area. It combines a reduced-calorie diet, behavior modification techniques, and an exercise program and is usually presented in weekly sessions for adolescents and their parents. A program using a similar approach, without the physical activity component, was studied in two randomized controlled trials published in the 1990s; it was found to be safe and produced significant weight loss over a six-month period. Sothern says the program has since been updated and a physical activity component added. The current version has not been tested in a randomized clinical trial. Of a group of 93 adolescents enrolled in the current program for a year, 56 agreed to be evaluated for a recent study. In that subset, participants had reduced their BMIs from an average of 32.3 at the program's start to an average of 28.2 at one year. (However, the results in the 37 adolescents who declined to be evaluated may have been quite different.) Longer-term follow-up data on Committed to Kids participants are not available.

In addition to programs that require regular attendance for a prescribed period, dozens of summer camps offer short-term treatment for overweight kids. However, few scientific studies have examined whether such camps work. Leonard Epstein points out that it's also difficult for families to evaluate commercial weight-loss programs or camps for children, since there are no laws requiring that such programs be scientifically evaluated for safety or effectiveness before they are marketed to the public. "Anybody can just say they have a program and start it," he says. He suggests that parents considering such a program should ask a series of questions: "I'd want to know how many families they have treated, the length of the program, and what kind of a BMI change or percent overweight change they usually get." He advises parents to ask about the staff's credentials, the program's dropout rate, and whether officials can provide any data on how well participants maintain their weight loss after the program ends. Parents may also find it helpful to talk with others whose children have attended. "I'd want a program that also took care of the parents," he adds. "I think family-based programs are always going to be better than programs that just target the child."

🐜🐜🐜

Prescription medicines to promote weight loss have had a checkered history, with dangerous side effects forcing some drugs to be taken off the market or to be prohibited for use as weight-loss aids. Amphetamines, considered safe for certain other uses, were once widely prescribed as diet pills but produced heart palpitations, high blood pressure, psychiatric symptoms, addiction, and other serious complications in some people who used them to induce weight loss; they are no longer approved for that purpose. Fenfluramine, prescribed during the 1990s as part of a popular two-drug weight-loss treatment nicknamed "fen-phen," was removed from the U.S. market after the combination was associated with heart valve damage in some users.

Nevertheless, the search continues for safer and more effective medicines to help people lose weight. Inspired by recent advances in scientific understanding of how the body regulates appetite and weight, researchers are currently pursuing a host of new drugs for treating obesity. Perhaps one or more of these candidates will turn out to be well-tailored medicines that can safely and specifically produce weight loss or help people avoid regaining lost pounds without undesirable side effects. At the moment, however, the drugs approved for treating obesity in adults are only modestly effective: used in combination with diet and exercise, they can help people lose a bit more weight than they would otherwise. Individual patients often benefit most during the early weeks of treatment, with the drugs becoming somewhat less effective over time. These medicines have side effects that make them inadvisable for some people to take. Only one is approved for use in children. Current treatment guidelines recommend that kids or teenagers should be prescribed weight-loss drugs only as an adjunct to better-established treatment strategies such as dietary modification, increased activity, and family therapy.

Two drugs—orlistat (Xenical) and sibutramine (Meridia)—are

approved for use in adults to aid in weight loss. Orlistat has recently been approved for obese children 12 years old or older. It does not suppress appetite, but it partially blocks the absorption of fat from the digestive tract, so that people on the drug do not fully digest and store all the fat calories they eat. In two studies on obese adolescents aged 12 to 16, children taking the drug reduced their BMI while those taking a placebo did not. In adult studies the drug improved weight loss in people on a weight-reducing diet and helped them maintain weight loss for up to two years. The drug's most common troublesome side effects are oily bowel movements and oily spotting on underwear caused by unabsorbed fat that ends up in the feces. Because it can interfere with the absorption of the soluble vitamins, people taking the drug must also take a daily supplement.

Sibutramine is an appetite suppressant that affects the functioning of nerve cells in the many brain pathways that use the chemical signals norepinephrine and serotonin. It can raise blood pressure and pulse rate and is hazardous for people with high blood pressure, various types of heart disease, or a history of stroke. In adult patients it produces moderate weight loss when combined with a calorie-restricted diet. In one large European study in adults, almost half of people who took the drug were able to maintain most of their weight loss for two years, compared with only 16 percent of people who took a placebo. However, a large number of participants dropped out of both groups, which limits the conclusions that can be drawn.

Robert Berkowitz conducted a trial of sibutramine in overweight teenagers. In his study kids who were given the drug in addition to standard obesity treatment lost about twice as much weight as those given a placebo, and most were able to keep the weight off for up to 12 months. They reported that sibutramine reduced hunger and made it easier for them to stick with their eating plan. Almost half of the teenagers taking the drug, however, experienced increases in blood pressure or pulse severe enough to require lowering the dose or in some cases stopping the medication. Experts caution that longer and larger studies are needed before the drug is approved for use in teenagers.

Overweight adolescents at risk of developing diabetes may benefit from a different drug, metformin (Glucophage). Approved as a treatment for type 2 diabetes in adults and in children 10 and older, metformin is not a weight-loss treatment, but in overweight adults with prediabetes it has been found to reduce the risk of developing diabetes or to delay the disease's onset. Some experts are also using it in overweight teenagers whose blood tests show a prediabetic pattern of abnormalities, such as high fasting insulin levels.

The best evidence supporting metformin's value in delaying diabetes comes from the Diabetes Prevention Program, a large government-funded clinical trial whose results have important health implications for millions of overweight Americans. Participants in the study—all of whom were at least 25 years old—were obese (average BMI: 34) and had impaired glucose tolerance, as shown by a high fasting blood glucose or an abnormal response to an oral glucose tolerance test. One group was assigned to intensive lifestyle changes to reduce weight and increase exercise, a second group was assigned to take metformin, and a third group was given a placebo and standard medical care. In the placebo group, 29 percent developed diabetes during the follow-up period, which averaged three years. In contrast, 14 percent of the lifestyle change group developed the disease (representing a 58 percent reduction in risk), and 22 percent of the metformin group developed diabetes (a 31 percent reduction in risk).

Metformin improves the body's control of glucose by increasing the liver's sensitivity to insulin and by reducing the liver's production of glucose. Unlike most other diabetes drugs, metformin does not promote weight gain. Its major risk is its potential for causing lactic acidosis, a rare but serious metabolic disorder that happens most often in people with kidney disease, liver disease, or heart failure—problems uncommon in children and teenagers.

Some doctors feel the Diabetes Prevention Program findings, combined with data from studies in adolescents, justify prescribing metformin for overweight teenagers who have impaired glucose tolerance, or prediabetes, although the drug is not currently approved for this purpose. Duke University researchers conducted a trial of metformin in obese children aged 12 to 19 who had high fasting insulin levels and found that the drug improved their insulin sensitivity and lowered both insulin levels and BMI. "Through its ability to reduce fasting blood glucose and insulin concentrations and to moderate weight gain, metformin might complement the effects of dietary and exercise counseling and reduce the risk of type 2 diabetes" in some patients, they write. Type 2 diabetes rates are rising dramatically as American kids become more overweight. The proven benefits of metformin for delaying diabetes in adults should make additional studies of its potential value for children with prediabetes an urgent priority.

What about nonprescription weight-loss aids? Consumers in general should steer clear of dietary supplements and over-the-counter (OTC) medicines that are promoted for weight loss. In particular, such products should not be used by children or adolescents. Unlike the prescription drugs described previously, a wide variety of herbal products and dietary supplements are aggressively marketed as weight-loss treatments with no requirement for approval by the Food and Drug Administration (FDA) and, therefore, no legal standards demanding scientific proof of their safety and efficacy. Ingredients of dietary supplements marketed for weight loss include chitosan, chromium picolinate, conjugated linoleic acid, and garcinia cambogia. Scientists reviewing the medical literature have found that there is insufficient data to show that any of these agents are safe or effective. "Because of the unpredictable amounts of active ingredients and the potential for harmful effects, the National Institutes of Health guidelines state that herbal preparations are not recommended as part of a weight-loss program," concludes a recent review by NIH scientists.

Some OTC medicines are also promoted to help people lose weight. Although the FDA regulates OTC drugs more stringently than it does dietary supplements, there is little evidence of their long-term effectiveness. Phenylpropanolamine, until recently a major ingredient in many OTC drugs sold as weight-loss remedies and nasal decongestants, was taken off the U.S. market after it was shown to increase the risk of strokes caused by bleeding in the brain. Ephedra and chemically related substances (known as ephedrine alkaloids, including the dietary supplement ma huang) have long been major ingredients in dietary supplements promoted for weight loss. They too have been linked with serious complications, including heart attacks, abnormal heart rhythms, strokes, seizures, and sudden deaths and were ordered off the market by the FDA in 2004. Ephedrine remains an approved ingredient in some OTC decongestants and asthma drugs.

🐾🐾🐾

On a soft spring day, Brian came home to Washington, D.C., from Cumberland Hospital, in southeastern Virginia, 104 pounds lighter than when he had been admitted as a patient eight months earlier. At 271 pounds Brian was still a heavyset young African American man, but he was no longer the nearly 400-pound teenager whose doctor had hospitalized him to lose weight because at 17 he had developed the kind of diabetes more often seen in overweight adults.

Cumberland is an isolated pediatric rehabilitation hospital set in marshy woodland, a place that specializes in slimming down children and teenagers whose obesity threatens their lives. The hospital once treated a 14-year-old who weighed 650 pounds; another patient was 12 years old, 5 feet tall, and weighed 500 pounds. Because specialized in-hospital treatment for obese kids is so difficult to find, patients have come from as far away as Alaska and Saudi Arabia. To the round-faced, homesick teenager from the District of Columbia, it felt like a prison. "I ain't going to lie," he says. "I thought I was in hell." Brian's obesity had been fueled by a voracious appetite. "My son could eat a whole pizza," recalled his mother, Cassandra. "He'd eat a box and a half of cereal in one day. A gallon of milk, he'd go through like nothing. Cookies, candy—he loved to eat."

In the hospital every aspect of Brian's life was transformed. For the early weeks of his stay he was placed on a regimen of medically monitored semistarvation called a protein-sparing modified fast. He was given a small amount of protein plus vitamin and mineral supplements and ample fluids each day so that his body was forced to break down fat rapidly to keep him alive. He lost about a pound a day. Staff members watched him constantly to make sure he didn't sneak food. Brian saw a psychotherapist several times a week and attended group sessions with other teenage patients to discuss the feelings and situations that could trigger his compulsive eating. He was taught how to read food labels and went on a field trip to learn what to order at

McDonald's. As he continued to lose weight, his doctors gradually liberalized his diet to allow him more calories and more choice about what he ate.

This type of inpatient treatment is only for children who are considered morbidly obese. They must be suffering medical complications serious enough to urgently threaten their health, and their doctors must determine that appropriate treatment in the community is either unavailable or unlikely to produce sufficiently rapid weight loss. Hospital director Daniel Davidow said the residential program at Cumberland, which also includes a daily exercise regimen, physical and occupational therapy, and a school program, costs between $800 and $1,000 per day. One boy who was at the hospital with Brian needed a heart transplant but was too heavy to undergo the operation. Others suffered from dangerous sleep apnea: their throats would close up as they slept and they would stop breathing. Some had legs so bowed from carrying excess pounds that they could scarcely walk. A few teenagers treated at Cumberland were being considered for gastric bypass surgery, an operation now being used to treat extreme obesity in adults, yet had been ordered by their surgeons to lose some weight before they could safely undergo the procedure.

Before he was judged ready to leave the hospital, Brian needed to reduce his BMI—which was initially above 55—to below 40. (Davidow explained that a BMI of 40 is considered the boundary between "severe clinical obesity" and "morbid obesity," according to guidelines for adults.) In addition, the Cumberland staff had to feel reasonably confident that Brian had acquired the skills and motivation to stick to the diet he would have to follow at home to maintain his weight loss. He was told that his future health depended on reaching those goals: if he regained the lost pounds, his diabetes would inevitably worsen, putting him at high risk of future heart disease, kidney failure, blindness, and other complications. A planned six-month stay stretched to eight. Brian celebrated his eighteenth birthday in the hospital. At last the day arrived for him to go home.

Brian and his mother were proud of what he achieved during his hospital stay, but for Brian the far bigger challenge was to keep the pounds off once he was back in his world—a world where fast food was plentiful, getting regular exercise was difficult, and everyday life was filled with the stresses of living with his single mother, struggling to finish high school, and trying to fit in among the other young men and women in his neighborhood. Within a month or two of his return to Washington, Brian had regained about 30 pounds of the weight he had lost, according to his former doctor at Washington's Children's National Medical Center. Now legally an adult, he told his mother he did not want to go back to his doctor—in fact, he didn't want to go to doctors at all anymore.

Dozens of studies have shown that maintaining weight loss is much harder than losing it, because the human body has evolved highly effective mechanisms to defend itself against starvation. Weight loss activates those defenses, even prompting the body to lower its resting metabolic rate and to make muscles work more efficiently so they burn less energy during physical activity.

Brian and the other children and teenagers who undergo weight-loss treatment at Cumberland Hospital are at the extreme end of the obesity curve—so heavy that their BMIs are literally off the growth charts and their bodies are being ravaged by the medical consequences of carrying so much fat. Such super-obese children are becoming more numerous in our society, and their treatment is a subject of intense debate. In many cases multiple biological and social factors combine to produce this degree of obesity. These children often come from families where virtually everyone is fat, families that have lost numerous loved ones to diseases caused by excess weight. There are super-obese kids who also have a history of overeating compulsively, sometimes for reasons in addition to hunger: to protect themselves from physical or sexual abuse, to assuage depression or anxiety. Some live in neighborhoods without supermarkets or recreational facilities, neighborhoods where high crime rates and gang activity make it dangerous for them to venture outside.

Hospital-based treatment programs like the one at Cumberland are rare. Despite their high cost, there is no evidence that they are any more effective than community-based outpatient programs for achieving long-term weight loss, says Thomas Wadden, a psychologist at the University of Pennsylvania who has reviewed research findings on treating obesity in children and teenagers. Very-low-calorie diets like the one Brian received during the initial weeks of his stay do produce rapid weight loss, often a pound or more per day, which is sometimes necessary for treating life-threatening complications of obesity. However, Wadden says, studies show that children or teenagers who lose weight on these diets usually regain at least half the weight lost within a year of stopping treatment.

Because of the high failure rate of medical treatments for severe obesity—especially among adolescents—small but growing numbers of very obese teenagers are undergoing the same kind of weight-loss surgery whose popularity has surged in recent years for obese adults. In the United States, the operation done most frequently to induce weight loss is called gastric bypass, but several other procedures are also being performed by surgeons in this country and abroad. An estimated 120,000 such operations were performed in the United States during 2003, and the number is expected to continue to grow.

Such operations, collectively known as bariatric surgery, are by far the most effective way doctors have discovered to produce long-lasting weight loss. Considered major surgery, in most cases they permanently alter the anatomy of the digestive tract. They carry a small risk of death at the time of operation (about 1 percent if the surgeon and hospital team are experienced in the procedure, but significantly higher if the surgeon and staff are not trained in bariatric surgery or have handled few such cases). They can cause short- and long-term complications. They are also expensive, typically $25,000 to $30,000. Insurance carriers have become so alarmed by the rapidly expanding cost of bariatric surgery that some have refused to pay for certain types of procedures and others have established criteria to strictly limit coverage even for severely obese adults with obesity-related medical problems.

In part, these operations are designed to force obese people to drastically reduce their intake of calories: one surgeon refers to them as "behavioral surgery." In addition to restricting stomach capacity, the procedures seem to reduce appetite, probably by altering the levels of various chemical messengers produced in the stomach and intestinal tract that influence perceptions of hunger and satiety. Because gastric bypass and some of the other bypass procedures also reduce the digestive tract's ability to absorb nutrients, including some vitamins and minerals, people become vulnerable to nutritional deficiencies for the rest of their lives. They must be willing to follow dietary instructions, take multiple pills daily, and see their doctors regularly. If they fail to take their daily supplements, they can develop anemia, bone disease, and many other problems.

Although some data currently exist on adults who have been living healthy lives following such surgery for 15 years, 20 years, or longer, they come chiefly from the "case series" of individual surgeons, not from randomized controlled trials that compared long-term outcomes in obese patients treated surgically with those who received standard nonsurgical treatment for their obesity and its complications. There are no studies yet on the surgery's long-term effects on teenagers, whose bodies are still developing and who can be expected to live for many decades after undergoing such operations. Medical experts are understandably nervous about the uncontrolled use of bariatric surgery in adolescents, yet surgeons who have studied the treatment's effects for years in their adult patients point out that the weight loss resulting from bariatric surgery usually cures or dramatically improves diabetes, high blood pressure, high cholesterol, sleep apnea, orthopedic problems, and numerous other complications of obesity. If serious medical problems are threatening an obese teenager's life they argue, why should such a patient be denied access to this surgery simply because he or she is not yet 18 years old?

During the past 25 years surgeons have devised several operations for producing weight loss. Because surgical procedures are not legally regulated the way drugs or medical devices are, different operations have proliferated without first being subjected to the kinds of studies required of medicines and without being scientifically compared with one another. In the United States the most frequent and most thoroughly studied bariatric operation is the Roux-en-Y gastric bypass, in which most of the stomach is closed off and a small stomach pouch is connected to the jejunum, the middle portion of the small intestine. The result is that food "bypasses" most of the stomach and the entire duodenum, the first part of the small intestine. This operation both restricts stomach capacity so that patients cannot eat much food at a time and reduces absorption of nutrients by the digestive tract. Gastric bypass operations can be done either as open surgery—through a large incision—or laparoscopically, which requires only a small incision.

In Israel, Australia, and much of Europe a more common operation is adjustable gastric banding, in which a surgeon, operating through a viewing device called a laparoscope, positions an inflatable belt or band around the upper portion of the stomach. A tube leads from the band to an external injection port on the abdominal wall. At any time after the operation doctors can inject saline solution through the tube to inflate the band, gradually restricting the diameter of the stomach so the patient will be able to eat only small amounts at a time. They can also remove saline to deflate the band if the diameter becomes too small, causing discomfort or nausea. Unlike gastric bypass surgery, adjustable gastric banding is easily reversible and doesn't involve cutting through the digestive tract or permanently altering its anatomy, and it's less likely to cause malabsorption of nutrients and lead to nutritional deficiencies. It is thus a lower-risk procedure. These advantages have led some experts to argue that it might be a more appropriate operation for severely obese adolescents, but in the United States the procedure is relatively new, and the band is currently approved for use only in patients 18 and older. Some U.S. trials of the device have reported significant complications with the adjustable band as well as lesser degrees of weight loss than with gastric bypass. Even in countries where the gastric band is widely used, long-term data on its success are not yet available; recipients have generally been monitored for less than a decade.

In studies of gastric bypass surgery during the past 10 years, about 10 percent of patients have suffered serious postoperative complications, including blood clots, bleeding, infections, problems with wound healing, bowel obstruction, and hernias. Both the risk of dying and the risk of complications are highly dependent on the surgeon's expertise and the number of such procedures routinely performed at the hospital. The chances of long-term complications from the operation are much more uncertain. Common problems include gallstones (which can be associated with rapid weight loss) and nutritional deficiencies such as iron-deficiency anemia, osteoporosis and fractures caused by calcium deficiency, and other diseases arising from vitamin deficiencies. One of the major questions about the operation's use in adolescents is whether its effect on absorption of calcium and other minerals will cause eventual weakening of bones. Moreover, the procedure is not uniformly successful. Most patients lose weight steadily for a year or two but then reach a plateau, and some regain the lost weight. In studies of more than 600 patients by surgeon Walter J. Pories, patients had lost, on average, almost 70 percent of their excess weight at one year after surgery. By 14 years after surgery they had kept off an average of about 50 percent of the original excess weight, but there was considerable individual variation.

Despite the operation's risks, there is some evidence that in severely obese adults it can improve health and may prolong life. Surgeon Kenneth G. MacDonald and colleagues compared outcomes in 154 obese adults with diabetes who had the surgery and 78 similar patients who did not undergo the procedure, either out of personal choice or because medical insurance would not pay for it. The annual chance of dying was 4.5 percent in patients who had not had the surgery, but only 1 percent in the surgical group. Pories found that in 83 percent of his obese patients with type 2 diabetes and in 99 percent of those with abnormal glucose tolerance, the operation cured the disorder, normalizing patients' blood levels of insulin and glucose. The weight loss produced by gastric bypass surgery also improves and sometimes normalizes high blood pressure, high cholesterol and triglycerides, heart function, and obesity-related liver disease. It commonly cures sleep apnea and pseudotumor cerebri, a potentially life-threatening obesity-related condition caused by elevated pressure of the fluid surrounding the brain. It improves weight-related respiratory and bladder problems. In women it often restores menstrual regularity and improves fertility and pregnancy outcomes. Losing large amounts of weight dramatically increases the ability of very obese people to move around, work, exercise, and perform routine daily tasks that most other people take for granted. At support group meetings for adults who have undergone the surgery, recipients often say that their operation marked the start of a new life.

In 1991 a panel of experts convened at a consensus development conference sponsored by the National Institutes of Health concluded that bariatric surgery could be considered an appropriate treatment for certain very obese adults, but that there were too few data to recommend the surgery for people under 18. The guidance expressed in the 1991 consensus statement is widely followed by the medical community and the insurance industry; nevertheless, in recent years it is likely (based on anecdotal evidence from bariatric surgeons) that more than 100 severely obese teenagers have undergone such operations.

Harvey J. Sugerman of Virginia Commonwealth University, a pioneer in the field of bariatric surgery, recently reviewed the results of gastric bypass surgery done at his hospital in 33 adolescents aged 12 to 18. Complication rates were similar to those seen in adults; there were no operative deaths. Two patients died suddenly two years and six years, respectively, after the procedure—probably of causes unrelated to the surgery, but the deaths are worrisome. Most patients lost weight successfully and kept off significant amounts, but five (about 15 percent) regained most or all the weight they had lost. Two additional "late deaths" in adolescents who had undergone weight-loss surgery were reported by pediatric surgeon C. W. Breaux of Birmingham, Alabama. These deaths occurred 15 months and 3 $^1/_2$ years, respectively, after the procedure.

When might bariatric surgery be medically and ethically justified in a teenager? Surgeons and obesity experts at Cincinnati Children's Hospital Medical Center have proposed a set of guidelines addressing this controversial question. Because the long-term balance of risks and benefits of this kind of surgery is so uncertain in adolescents, they urge that whenever such operations are contemplated for people under 18, the patients should be evaluated and treated at medical centers that offer comprehensive childhood obesity treatment and by a skilled surgical team that is committed to collecting detailed data and performing careful follow-up on all patients. (In the United States that is not the case at present: many bariatric surgeons around the country operate occasionally on adolescents without systematically collecting information on outcomes.)

Victor F. Garcia, the pediatric surgeon who founded the Cincinnati program, believes strongly that surgery should not be denied to adolescents whose obesity is causing them serious medical problems and who have been unable to lose weight by other means. He argues, however, that bariatric surgery in children under 18 should be regionalized and performed only at centers that can offer patients a surgeon experienced in such procedures, a multidisciplinary support team, and a commitment to providing long-term follow-up care and collecting data on outcomes. He points to cancer treatment in children as a specialty that has been successfully regionalized and could provide a model for bariatric surgery in obese adolescents. "I fear that unless it is regionalized . . . we are going to have children unnecessarily undergoing surgery, suffering complications and even dying," Garcia says.

The Cincinnati physicians propose in their guidelines that BMI criteria for considering surgery in people under 18 should be more stringent than in adults. The 1991 consensus document indicates that adults with a BMI above 40 may be considered potential candidates for bariatric surgery, as well as certain patients with BMIs between 35 and 40 who are suffering severe medical complications of their obesity. However, they suggest that in adolescents the surgery should be considered only for patients with a BMI of 40 or higher who have serious medical complications of obesity, such as diabetes, sleep apnea, or pseudotumor cerebri. It could also be considered in those with a BMI of 50 or higher who have less serious complications, including severe psychosocial difficulties related to obesity, if weight loss is likely to correct such problems. They emphasize that decisions about surgery should be made on an individual basis, primarily by considering the impact of obesity on health rather than relying on absolute BMI cutoffs. They recommend that adolescents should not be considered for surgery unless they have failed to lose weight during at least six months of organized attempts at weight management, as determined by their primary doctors. Surgery also should not be considered unless an adolescent has attained at least 95 percent of his or her predicted adult height, which usually occurs by about age 13 in girls and about age 15 in boys. An X-ray of the hand and wrist can indicate whether a child's bones still have significant growth to complete.

The Cincinnati guidelines also recommend that obese youngsters being considered for surgical treatment undergo a comprehensive psychological and medical evaluation. Factors precluding surgery would include a medically correctable cause of obesity; a history of recent substance abuse; pregnancy, breastfeeding, or plans for pregnancy in the near future; a medical, mental, or psychiatric condition that impairs the patient's ability to make an informed decision, to consent to surgery, or to follow doctors' instructions afterward; and an unwillingness or inability (on the part of the patient or family) to participate in regular checkups after the operation. Young people who have exhibited self-destructive behavior or who have been unable to stick with a medical regimen in the past are not considered good candidates for surgery.

Thomas H. Inge, surgical director of the Comprehensive Weight Management Center at Cincinnati Children's Hospital Medical Center and a coauthor of the guidelines, estimates that a quarter-million adolescents in the United States have a BMI of 40 or higher. Most of them have some medical or psychological consequences of their weight, including risk factors for diabetes or heart disease, but not all have developed obesity-related diseases. At the same time, as Inge and his coauthors acknowledge in the article describing their guidelines, the long-term metabolic, nutritional, and psychological effects of bariatric surgery in teenagers are unknown, and "the durability of surgically induced weight loss among adolescents remains to be clearly defined." He says, "It's easier for me to envision the risk/benefit ratio being in favor of the operation if the BMI is over 50." If a teenager's BMI were between 40 and 50 but the patient had no overt illness caused by being overweight, "I would hesitate," he adds. "They are adolescents, and we really need to be treating disease, not risk factors."

The Cincinnati surgeons are part of a multispecialty program devoted to treating obesity in children. Before proceeding with surgery, team members meet on several occasions with the patient and family to teach them what to expect. They require their adolescent patients to take a written test to evaluate how much they understand.

Each young candidate for surgery is then assessed by a panel that includes the surgeon, another physician who specializes in medical treatment of obesity, a child psychologist, and a dietitian. Panel members consider the medical issues, the child's ability to make decisions and cooperate with treatment, and the family environment. Between 2001 and the spring of 2004, 32 adolescents underwent gastric bypass surgery at Cincinnati Children's Hospital. The average age was 17 for girls and 16 for boys; the youngest patient was a 14-year-old girl with diabetes. The patients had an average BMI of 56, and all had obesity-related illnesses. Doctors are still studying the long-term outcome of the treatment in these young people.

Inge says that medical insurance has paid for surgery in some obese teenagers treated in the Cincinnati program. But with 23 million U.S. adults and a quarter-million U.S. adolescents who are overweight enough to be considered possible candidates, the potential demand for such surgery is great enough to overwhelm the nation's pool of trained surgeons and qualified hospitals. Bariatric surgeons in many cities have long waiting lists of obese adult patients. Most surgical residency programs have not yet developed the capacity to thoroughly impart the skills needed for bariatric surgery, especially for the newer laparoscopic techniques, and surgeons entering the field should attend training courses at qualified institutions before they embark on bariatric procedures. Anyone considering whether to have a gastric bypass or other weight-loss operation should be sure to obtain detailed information about the operating surgeon's experience and outcomes, as well as the volume of such cases performed at the hospital involved. "No matter how renowned the children's hospital is, make sure they have a surgeon who is experienced and well trained in doing the procedure," says pediatrician Victor Garcia. "If the surgeon doing this surgery has done only one, you are, I think, inviting disaster."

CHAPTER 9

Action for Healthy Communities

M aybe you and your kids are already on the right track. Your own eating habits are good, and you have acquired the skills and the resources to become an adept food shopper, stocking your kitchen with healthy items your children enjoy. You are physically active and enjoy playing vigorous games with your family and spending time with them walking, biking, and swimming. You keep track of what your children eat for lunch at school, and as a PTA member you've been active in improving the school's snack and drink offerings. You try to limit the amount of time your kids spend watching television or sitting at the computer. You figure you're doing just about all you can to prevent your family from becoming overweight. But what about your neighbors' children? What about your coworkers and their families? What about the other children in your community?

In Chapter 1, I told the story of Bruce, an overweight teenager who developed high blood pressure. Bruce's mother, Lottie, recognized that in order to help her son she needed to change the behavior of her entire family. She and her kids gave up habits they had previously considered "normal," like buying large botttles of regular soda and eating pizza several times a week. They adopted a new definition of normal that included eating more vegetables for dinner, watching less television, drinking more water or diet soda, and going for walks together around the track at the high school. Actions like Lottie's are what our nation needs on a grand scale. If the epidemic of childhood obesity is to be halted, large social changes are required. They will not happen unless people who care about children's health are willing to become active at the community, state, or national level, working to create a healthier environment for kids by changing social policies.

Major economic forces—among them food manufacturers, restaurant chains, automobile makers, real estate developers, and the entertainment industry—have strong financial interests in maintaining various aspects of the status quo. No single one of these industries or sectors deserves the blame for our nation's obesity epidemic, but together, many of their products and services (and the ways they are marketed) have contributed to Americans' unhealthy lifestyle. Each of these groups has political clout that it can bring to bear on government officials to oppose policy changes that are against its own interests. That is one reason why many obesity experts believe that it will take determined, well-organized efforts by concerned citizens and advocacy groups to bring about health-promoting change in our communities and our nation. "Indeed, it is difficult to think of any major industry that might benefit if people ate less food; certainly not the agriculture, food product, grocery, restaurant, diet, or drug industries," writes nutrition professor Marion Nestle of New York University. "All flourish when people eat more, and all employ armies of lobbyists to discourage governments from doing anything to inhibit overeating."

Psychologist and nutrition activist Kelly D. Brownell of Yale University coined the phrase "the toxic environment" to refer to the many factors in American society that combine to promote unhealthy weight gain. He believes that grassroots action offers the best hope of detoxifying that environment. "If we ask whether this obesity problem is going to be won from the top down or from the bottom up, it's very clear," Brownell recently told an audience at the Johns Hopkins Bloomberg School of Public Health. "Very little is happening at the top. A lot is happening at the bottom." An Institute of Medicine report,

Preventing Childhood Obesity: Health in the Balance, urges Americans to recognize the need to work together to combat this urgent threat to our children's health. "Preventing childhood obesity should become engrained as a collective responsibility," the report states. Individuals, families, communities, corporations, and governments must all accept some share of the task of meeting this challenge.

But what should a concerned citizen do? Obesity is a dominant topic in the news media these days, and the cacophony of advice and policy initiatives issuing from health officials, politicians, and activists often seems overwhelming. From a "junk food tax" to mandatory nutrition labels on restaurant menus, from reform of federal policies on farm subsidies to required daily physical education classes in schools, state and federal legislators have proposed hundreds of bills offering possible remedies. Many of the policies being considered represent strategies for changing our shared environment. Giving each family the knowledge and skills needed to develop healthier habits is certainly desirable, but realistically, even if families become better informed about how to improve kids' diets and encourage them to be physically active, this may not be sufficient to prevent the spread of obesity among our children. Changing our common environment in ways that will foster healthier food choices and greater access to physical activity is likely to have a broader and more rapid impact.

In this chapter I try to provide some guidance to readers who want to work to prevent obesity in their communities or to become politically active on issues related to childhood obesity at the state or national level. I have already discussed school food policies and physical education programs in previous chapters, so I will not do so again here, although these may be areas where many parents will want to focus their efforts first. After some general suggestions about how to get started, I will offer more specific points of contact for three possible areas of action: the growing movement to limit or regulate food and drink advertising that targets children; efforts to make neighborhoods more walkable and bikeable and to increase other local opportunities for physical activity; and strategies to increase access to fresh and healthy foods in underserved communities, which include many low-income urban neighborhoods and rural areas.

EXPLORE THE LOCAL POLITICAL SCENE

If you have children in a public school, you may already have talked with others in your community—parents, teachers, a principal, or a school nurse—who are concerned about the obesity epidemic and about children's health. These people can serve as your initial contacts. Your pediatrician or family physician may also be able to tell you about local community efforts to combat obesity. Find out whether a childhood obesity task force has been formed in your city or town. Such committees are being established in many communities and typically include representatives from the health department, school system, parks and recreation department, PTA, public transportation department, and other organizations such as consumer groups working on issues of zoning, bike lanes, and sidewalks for pedestrian safety. At task force meetings, people with different areas of expertise can share information and come up with a range of ideas for improving the situation in their city or town. Probably the best way to find out whether such a task force exists in your area is to contact your local health department.

Read the newspaper and check the Web sites of local and state governments to learn whether your elected representatives have sponsored any programs or legislation related to childhood obesity. Let elected officials know of your concern about this issue. Contact community organizations that may be working on the topic, such as food banks or the YMCA. If there is a school of public health in your city or town, researchers there may be studying strategies to reduce obesity in the surrounding community.

Scores of bills addressing various aspects of the obesity epidemic are introduced in state legislatures each year. Nonprofit organizations working on obesity-related issues have found that legislators are especially likely to respond when contacted by constituents who can cite statistics indicating a possible link between specific health problems—such as a high local prevalence of childhood obesity, adult diabetes, or high blood pressure—and local conditions in the community, such as a shortage of supermarkets or safe places to play.

The Web sites listed on page 271 in Resources may provide helpful information on a range of obesity-related policy initiatives.

REDUCE THE UNHEALTHY IMPACT OF
CHILD-TARGETED ADVERTISING

The advertising and marketing of products to American children have increased dramatically during the past two decades, with foods, beverages, and fast food restaurants accounting for the lion's share of products and services promoted to kids. Nutrition researchers estimate that food and beverage advertisers currently spend between $10 billion and $12 billion each year to reach children and youth, partly in an effort to get children to buy their products, but also because demands from children can greatly influence the purchasing decisions of adults. In 2002 annual sales of foods and drinks to children and adolescents in the United States totaled more than $27 billion.

Much of the promotion of foods, drinks, toys, and other products to children takes place on television. The average American child now sees an estimated 40,000 television commercials each year, twice as many as during the 1970s. Reviewing the past decade's research on child-targeted TV advertising for its report on preventing childhood obesity, a panel of experts assembled by the Institute of Medicine concluded that "more than 50 percent of television advertisements directed at children promote foods and beverages such as candy, fast food, snack foods, soft drinks, and sweetened breakfast cereals that are high in calories and fat, low in fiber, and low in nutrient density." Children see one food commercial, on average, during every five minutes of television that they watch. Athletes and pop stars admired by kids receive lucrative contracts to endorse products and to appear in food, soda, or restaurant commercials. Foods are also increasingly marketed to children through strategic "product placement" on television shows and in children's movies, video games, and interactive Web sites. In this strategy the product literally becomes part of the story or game: often a popular actor or a video character is shown eating the food being promoted.

Children are also exposed to food, drink, and restaurant advertising in schools. Channel One, a daily broadcast that reaches an estimated eight million teenage students in more than 350,000 classrooms throughout the United States shows 10 minutes of news and 2 minutes of commercials each day; schools receive free video equipment in exchange for requiring students to watch the program. In a study conducted during a four-week period in the early 1990s, researchers found that more than two-thirds of Channel One's commercials were for food products, including fast food, soft drinks, chips, and candy. Candy, cereal, and pizza makers also offer schools free "educational materials" featuring math or science lessons that use their products, and some donut, pizza, and fast food chains offer academic incentives that include free food for students with good records for attendance, behavior, or homework completion.

Although advertisers maintain that the purpose of advertising food products to children is to attract them to specific brands rather than to influence their diet as a whole, studies clearly show that food advertising prompts children to nag their parents to buy heavily advertised products, and some evidence indicates that it also affects their overall consumption of various categories of foods and beverages. Advertising's specific impact on children's diets has been difficult to quantify because so many factors influence food choices. After reviewing the available research, the IOM panel of obesity experts concluded that the effects of advertising "are unlikely to be limited to brand choice. Wider impacts include the increased consumption of energy-dense foods and beverages and greater engagement in sedentary behaviors, both of which contribute to energy imbalance and obesity."

Young children lack the thinking skills needed to evaluate an advertisement's claims. Child development research indicates that before the age of about 7 or 8, they don't even understand that the purpose of an advertisement is to persuade, rather than to entertain or to inform. For this reason, the American Academy of Pediatrics in 1995 issued a policy statement saying that "advertising directed toward children is inherently deceptive and exploits children under 8 years of age." Advertising industry executives apparently share some of the medical profession and the public's concerns about marketing products to very young children. In a 2004 poll of youth marketers conducted by Harris Interactive, 61 percent of respondents agreed with the statement that "advertising to children begins at too young an age."

Some advocacy groups have called for a federal ban on all advertising directed at children younger than 8 years old. Others are urging

Congress to reauthorize the Federal Trade Commission (FTC) to regulate advertising and marketing to children, as well as calling for an end to marketing in schools and for restrictions on the advertising to children of foods high in fat, sugar, and total calories. "There's no question that the current marketing practices take unfair advantage of children and are exploiting them," says Susan Linn, an instructor in psychiatry at Harvard Medical School and a leader of the Campaign for a Commercial-Free Childhood (CCFC), a coalition of groups advocating restrictions on marketing to kids. "We have to take it on as a societal issue."

The FTC's mandate includes regulating advertising to ensure that it is not unfair or deceptive. The agency tried once before, in 1978, to use that authority to restrict television advertising to children, on the grounds that all advertising that is directed at children too young to understand an ad's intent is inherently unfair and deceptive. Responding to fierce opposition to the proposed ban by the business community, Congress passed a law in 1980 withdrawing the FTC's authority to restrict children's advertising and prohibiting it from adopting the proposed rules. A renewed effort by the FTC to limit advertising to children would likely suffer from the same drawbacks as the 1970s effort, in terms of being impractical, ineffective, and likely unconstitutional, FTC associate director Mary K. Engle told the IOM expert panel at a workshop held in 2003. "The FTC is not a public health agency" but a law enforcement agency, Engle told the committee. To issue new rules restricting advertising to children, the FTC would have to be able to point to research indicating a direct link between the marketing of certain products to kids and an increase in childhood obesity and, furthermore, demonstrate that the proposed restrictions would substantially alleviate the obesity problem. In addition, advertisers would be likely to challenge any marketing restrictions in court. Engle noted that the U.S. Supreme Court has ruled in recent years that the government should attempt to limit free speech (which includes advertising) only as a last resort. Advertisers have already signaled their intention to fight any proposed action by Congress or the FTC. "As an industry, we strongly reject the claims that advertising causes childhood obesity and the related premise that new government restrictions or bans on advertising to children should be imposed," said Bob Liodice, chief executive of the Association of National Advertisers, in a statement quoted in the *Wall Street Journal.*

As an interim strategy, CCFC and some other advocacy groups have called on advertisers to establish a more vigorous system for policing the ways they market products to children. The current system of self-regulation is completely voluntary and relies on the Children's Advertising Unit, or CARU, a body established in 1974 by the industry-supported National Advertising Review Council. With a staff of only six full-time employees, CARU is charged with monitoring advertising to children in all media and responding to consumer complaints—a seemingly impossible task for such a small agency.

In its report the IOM panel concluded that even though advertising to children under the age of 8 is inherently unfair, "there is presently insufficient causal evidence that links advertising directly with childhood obesity and that would support a ban on all food advertising directed to children." The report also says that such a ban might not be feasible because of legal concerns about freedom of speech. It calls instead for the development of new, tougher guidelines that would be voluntarily implemented by the advertising industry. The report also recommends that the FTC be empowered to monitor the industry's compliance with the new guidelines, thus leaving open the possibility of government regulation in the future if the industry fails to cooperate. However, considering advertisers' record of strenuously opposing any limitations on marketing to kids, it seems unlikely that they will dramatically change their practices unless they encounter strong public or political pressure to do so.

Meanwhile, what can people do about marketing to children that they believe is harmful? They can and should monitor the content of the shows, ads, and movies their children watch, the video games they play, and other forms of entertainment, staying alert for product placements embedded in the film, show, or game. They can express their concerns both to marketers and to their own elected representatives. As consumers, they certainly can also complain to CARU about practices they feel are unfair or deceptive. Parents should find out whether Channel One and other sources of advertising are present in their local schools, and they can urge school officials, as the IOM report recommends, to make schools "advertising-free to the greatest possible extent." Parents and teachers can make a point of talking with kids about how advertising works, helping children to critically examine specific commercials or advertisements and to identify how ads try to persuade the viewer. They can also urge schools to include lessons on "media literacy" in their curricula, teaching kids to become more knowledgeable and skeptical users of media.

People concerned about marketing to children can monitor the progress of legislation and other proposals at the federal and state levels and can add their voices to the public debate either individually or through advocacy groups. Doug Wood, a New York–based attorney for the advertising industry, predicted in a recent interview with an online investors' newsletter that the National Association of Attorneys General might be more likely than the FTC to take legal action to restrict marketing to kids. He cited the association's successful suit several years ago against tobacco companies, in which the companies agreed as part of a settlement to stop marketing their products in ways that would appeal to children. Voters interested in that strategy might consider contacting their state attorney general.

On page 272 in Resources you'll find a partial list of organizations and Web sites that can provide further information on marketing to children and on the possible links between advertising and the obesity epidemic.

WALKABLE NEIGHBORHOODS WITH PLACES TO PLAY

The typical American suburb seems designed to discourage physical activity. Many developments are built without sidewalks or crosswalks. Schools, especially recently built ones, are often large complexes on multiacre sites located on the periphery of neighborhoods, frequently on major roads with heavy traffic. Shops, libraries, cafes, and markets are often several miles from people's homes, difficult or impossible to reach on foot or by public transportation. Parks, playgrounds, and community centers also may not be within convenient or safe walking distance. People living in such neighborhoods often feel they have "no place to walk to." Whenever they want to go somewhere, they are forced to go by car. Studies suggest that the layout of such communities is contributing to the obesity epidemic. People who live in mixed-use neighborhoods with access to shops and public transportation tend to walk more, and to weigh less, than those who live in sprawling, auto-mobile-dependent suburbs. The realization that people's body weight and overall health are influenced by the "built environment" is one factor behind the "smart growth" movement, which favors planning new development in ways that both protect the environment and cre-ate communities whose local resources are easily accessible on foot and by public transportation.

Most of us cannot easily change where we live, but there may be things we can do to make our communities more walkable and to im-prove local opportunities for physical activity available to children. In Charlottesville, Virginia, one of the first projects launched by the city's newly formed task force on childhood obesity after it began work in 1999 was the establishment of regular "walk-to-school" days in some neighborhoods. The suggestion came from a parent who knew about the national Safe Routes to School Programs, a collection of commu-nity-based efforts to make it possible for more of America's children to walk or ride their bicycles to school. On the first Friday of every month, children and parents were encouraged to walk to school. A local hospi-tal paid for some of the initial expenses, such as hiring extra crossing guards. The health department gave a bandanna to each child who participated. A volunteer from a local transportation advocacy organi-zation taught lessons to middle school students on pedestrian and bi-cycle safety in urban and suburban neighborhoods. Children who had to ride the bus on walk-to-school day took a walk around the track when they arrived, accompanied by their teachers. Parents were sur-veyed about available walking routes in their neighborhoods, and their suggestions about improving crosswalks at certain intersections were passed on to the city council.

The Charlottesville walk-to-school program is expanding to addi-tional schools and has generated demand for road improvements that will make the city's neighborhoods more walkable for everyone. Other communities around the nation report similar results from walk-to-school programs. Parents who are fearful at first of letting their children walk to school will often accept the idea of a "walking school bus," in which several adult volunteers walk a large group of children to school. Many parents become enthusiastic about walk-to-school programs and begin agitating for traffic lights, sidewalks, speed bumps, and bike lanes or paths to make streets safer for pedestrians and cyclists. A Safe Routes to School program can help provide the motivation for "retrofitting" an existing community to make it more walkable and bikeable. In California's Marin County, the percentage of children walking or biking to school increased from 21 percent when the program started to 38 percent two years later. Page 275 in Resources contains helpful information sources for people interested in starting a Safe Routes to School program.

As physical activity expert James Sallis points out, decisions about where to locate schools in neighborhoods are a key factor in determining walkability. "Nothing is going to substitute for organizing schools so that they're not on the periphery," he says. "They really need to be in the middle of communities, planned so that it's easy to walk and bike there. . . . Parents need to advocate for these sorts of things."

In a report issued in 2000, the nonprofit National Trust for Historic Preservation found that state and local policies often work against the preservation of small or historic neighborhood schools. State education departments may require or recommend unnecessarily large acreage standards for school sites, forcing towns to close existing schools and to build larger ones on the edges of the community, where land is more easily available. State and local governments do not always provide adequate funding for routine school maintenance, and building codes are sometimes biased toward new school construction rather than renovation or upgrading of existing schools. School districts are exempt from zoning and planning laws in many states, and real estate developers sometimes donate parcels of land in new subdivisions to the school district, thereby increasing the value of lots in the subdivision but also influencing policies on school location. If local residents educate themselves about zoning and school district policies, they can become advocates for the preservation of existing schools and the optimal planning and location of new schools.

Community residents can take other steps to make their neighborhoods more walkable and bikeable. On page 274 in Resources, I list organizations and Web sites that can provide suggestions, tools, and training.

Another important focus for activism to reduce childhood obesity rates is improving children's access to local recreational facilities and making sure that opportunities for physical activity are available after school. Once school is dismissed for the day, children in the United States spend the hours until dinnertime in a bewildering variety of settings. Some attend publicly or privately funded after-school programs, often at a local school or community center, where the primary focus is often on sitting and doing homework. Some go home to a parent, a relative, a babysitter, or an empty house or apartment. Some go to a licensed child-care center or family child-care facility. Some stay at school for sports practices or extracurricular activities. Part-time jobs, private sports leagues and teams, lessons and tutoring programs are also among the many other possibilities.

James Sallis considers the after-school hours a prime time for building more physical activity into children's day. There's no simple way for school or health officials to make this happen, though, because after-school care is so varied and decentralized. Pressure from parents and from other knowledgeable adults is the best way to change community norms to ensure that kids have the chance to play outside and to be physically active after school. Community activists can help both by raising awareness of the importance of physical activity among providers of after-school care and by taking inventory of the kinds of programs and recreational facilities available to children. In Charlottesville, members of the city's childhood obesity task force conducted a survey of more than 900 children in the fifth through eighth grades to find out what kinds of activities interested them and compared their responses with what was offered. They learned that the city's African American children wanted to take classes in hip-hop dancing; the girls also expressed interest in roller skating and cheerleading and the boys in basketball and wrestling. These activities either were not being offered or were not sufficient to meet the demand—for example, P.E. teachers did not feel qualified to teach dance, and local schools and playgrounds did not have enough basketball hoops. The Charlottesville task force has since formed a separate physical activity subcommittee that includes the city's director of parks and recreation. The subcommittee plans to survey after-school programs and sports leagues about their current offerings and to see what activities can be introduced or expanded. Some of its efforts will also focus on improving opportunities for children who are considered at high risk of becoming obese because they are already overweight, because they live in low-income neighborhoods with few recreational facilities, or because they do not consider themselves athletic.

An alternative strategy for mobilizing community and political support is to map a city or town's recreational opportunities and identify the gaps. In the Play Across Boston project, researchers from the Harvard School of Public Health and Northeastern University conducted a comprehensive, community-based assessment of parks, playgrounds, recreation centers, and other exercise facilities available to Boston's youth. They found that girls participated in sports and activity programs only half as often as boys and that African American and Hispanic youth were underserved relative to their share of the city's population. They also identified some significant and sometimes unexpected disparities in sports and recreational facilities among the city's neighborhoods. The Play Across Boston project provides a "playbook" of what the city can do to improve the activity environment for its children and reduce their risk of obesity, said Steven Gortmaker, one of the researchers who led the project. Similar playbooks could be compiled for other cities and towns across America.

See page 274 in Resources for information on initiatives to promote physical activity in communities.

BETTER FOOD CHOICES FOR ALL

American communities do not offer everyone equal access to healthy foods. Supermarkets and grocery stores are more plentiful in suburbs and in high-income neighborhoods; low-income enclaves in urban areas are much less likely to have supermarkets and well-stocked grocery stores, and residents of such areas may not own cars or have easy access to a supermarket via public transportation. This is why people in poor urban neighborhoods often must rely on convenience stores and fast food restaurants. The choices available in these settings are usually processed foods and meals or snack products high in calories, sugars, and unhealthy fats; there may be few fresh fruits and vegetables or whole grain items for sale. Many rural residents face a similar shortage of local grocery outlets. Ironically, despite our country's unequaled agricultural productivity, researchers have designated large swaths of the rural United States as "food deserts" because supermarkets and grocery stores are so sparse. Finding ways to make healthy food choices available to everyone should be a central part of our efforts to combat the epidemic of childhood obesity.

It's easy to see why supermarket companies might want to locate stores in high-income suburbs, but income differences don't fully explain why grocery stores and supermarkets are so unevenly distributed in American communities. The flight of supermarkets from city centers to suburbs began in the 1960s. In recent decades, as stores have grown in size, they have developed a format best adapted to areas offering large tracts of land and a relatively homogeneous population of consumers who can drive to the grocery store. In rural areas companies try to maximize sales and reduce overhead by increasingly locating their stores in large "supercenter" outlets, which many rural residents must drive long distances to reach. Sociologist Troy C. Blanchard of Mississippi State University has found that, in at least half of all nonmetropolitan U.S. counties not located adjacent to a large city, residents do not have ready access to a supermarket.

Although people's food purchases are undoubtedly influenced by food costs, there is also evidence that the types of food outlets available in neighborhoods influence local residents' diets and may affect their risk of obesity and of diet-related diseases. North Carolina researchers used census and survey data from several states to examine possible links between dietary intake and the local "food environment," including supermarkets, small grocery stores, convenience stores, fast food restaurants, and full-service restaurants. They found that, particularly for African Americans, living in a census tract with a supermarket was associated with a healthier diet in terms of fruits and vegetables, total fat, and saturated fat—and this association seemed to be independent of participants' level of income and education. There was even a "dose-response" effect: African Americans' intake of fruits and vegetables increased by 32 percent for each additional supermarket located in their census tract. A similar although smaller dose-response effect of supermarkets on fruit and vegetable intake was also seen for white Americans.

Health researchers and activists in some communities have used the implications of findings like these to launch ambitious efforts to improve the local food environment. One of the most exciting such projects is under way in Philadelphia. There, the Food Trust, a local nonprofit organization, issued a comprehensive report in 2001 that mapped the locations of supermarket sales within the city and compared them with a map of mortality rates from diet-related diseases. The report found that supermarkets were very unevenly distributed, with low-income areas particularly underserved. Within the most underserved sections of the city there were pockets where residents had especially high mortality rates from diet-related diseases, and these neighborhoods were designated as the areas with the greatest need. After the report's publication, Philadelphia's city council asked the Food Trust to help form a food marketing task force to address the problem of supermarket access. The group included representatives from the supermarket industry, city government, the financial sector, the real estate industry, and other members of the business community, as well as charities and community nonprofits. The task force recommendations included urging the city to target areas for new supermarkets, assist in finding parcels of land, and reduce regulatory barriers to investment. State government was also asked to establish a financing program to support local supermarket development.

The issue attracted the support of key state legislators from Philadelphia and Pittsburgh, who saw supermarkets as a source of jobs as well as a way of improving the health of city residents. In 2004 the state legislature appropriated $100 million for planning and low-interest loans to aid in supermarket development in underserved areas. Although politicians and activists have successfully fought for new supermarkets in other cities in the past, Pennsylvania's action represents the first time a state has put substantial public funding into supermarket development, according to Hannah Burton of the Food Trust. Burton said that planners hope to open four new supermarkets in Philadelphia within two years. Burton adds that a critical ingredient in Philadelphia's success was bringing representatives of various sectors together on the task force and getting them to work cooperatively. "They each contributed a piece of the answer," she says. Representatives of the supermarket industry, initially skeptical about the potential market for their stores in the target areas, became eager participants in the process.

Burton notes that community activists in other cities can pursue a similar strategy by trying to bring together local government officials, economic development groups, and representatives of the supermarket industry. The Food Trust found that providing mortality data for specific neighborhoods from diet-related diseases helped impress Philadelphia residents and their elected representatives with the importance of access to healthy foods. "You have to give people a reason to be interested in the issue. We found the public health data to be very important," Burton says. "We were able to cite specific addresses" for each diet-related disease death.

Concerned citizens can also work to change the local food environment on a smaller scale. An approach being tried in several locations is the Healthy Stores program, in which researchers and local activists work with food stores to increase the availability of healthy foods on shelves and promote their purchase. Public health researcher Joel Gittelsohn of the Johns Hopkins Center for Human Nutrition, in Baltimore, has conducted such programs in the Marshall Islands and on two Apache reservations in Arizona and is starting Healthy Stores programs in inner-city Baltimore, in Canada, and in Hawaii. In each case public health researchers work with store owners and with members of the local community to determine what kinds of healthy food options could be offered and marketed. When introducing new foods, workers in each local Healthy Stores program promote them with posters, cooking demonstrations, and taste tests to try to make sure they are accepted. "A lot can be done, but it takes time to work in stores," Gittelsohn points out. "Their primary motivation is to remain profitable. We're not there to make them lose money. They have to be convinced of that."

Another way to boost the local availability of fresh fruits and vegetables is to establish a farmers market. Many states, as well as the USDA, offer assistance in planning, developing, and operating farmers markets. Grant money may also be available. The number of farmers markets in the United States increased by more than 75 percent between 1994 and 2002 and currently totals more than 3,100. Local nutrition advocacy organizations in many areas have established such markets in urban neighborhoods and other settings.

The Food Trust offers suggestions for anyone interested in developing an outdoor farmers market:

- Find a site with good visibility from streets and walkways, such as a park or a shaded parking lot. "It should be a frequently traveled location, someplace where people are going past," says the Food Trust's Brian Lang.
- Find a sponsor, such as a local community organization or redevelopment agency. Such agencies may be able to provide some money to help pay for start-up costs.
- Get permission from the local government and the support of local elected officials.
- Recruit farmers through the state department of agriculture, farmers organizations, 4-H clubs, or local nutrition advocacy groups. Lang has found that publishing a listing or advertisement in a local newspaper or farming newsletter is an especially efficient way to recruit. The Food Trust asks participating farmers to pay a market fee that is between 3 percent and 5 percent of sales to help defray the cost of administering the market.
- Establish procedures to ensure an efficient and orderly market, such as requirements for participation, types of products to be sold, and signage. You may be able to get local real estate developers or redevelopment agencies to pay for permanent signs announcing the market's location and schedule.
- Once your market is ready to open, advertise it in the local newspaper and send out press releases to get local media to run news

stories about it. "Often, sales will lag for one or two months and eventually a community newspaper will do a story," Lang says. "There's a noticeable difference in the number of people there the next week."

On page 275 in Resources you'll find a list of organizations and Web sites offering information on becoming involved in improving your local food environment.

The childhood obesity epidemic has its roots in many aspects of our biology and modern lifestyle. It threatens the future health of millions of children, not just in our own country but around the world. And because it is a problem that has been decades in the making, overcoming it—if indeed that is possible—will take decades as well. If obesity rates continue to rise on the trajectory they have followed in recent years, the epidemic and its inevitable medical consequences will impair the health and shorten the lives of today's children and of those yet to be born.

Americans have seen heartening evidence, in the recent history of our nation's relationship with tobacco, that large-scale social, political, and behavioral change is possible. We all have a part to play in combating the obesity epidemic. The more we learn about the fascinating interplay of biology, environment, and behavior that governs the human body's control of appetite and body weight, the greater will be our chances of helping our children maintain a healthy weight. The better we, as consumers and citizens, understand the factors within modern American society that influence our personal food and activity choices, the more we will become empowered to transform our shared environment into one that no longer produces a nation of ever-fatter children.

Resources

T he books, publications, and Web sites listed in this section provide a starting point for readers who want to learn more about
many of the topics covered in this book. It is impossible for
any source list on childhood obesity to be comprehensive, but I have
mentioned sources that I found valuable in my research and others
that experts have recommended.

OBESITY AND ITS HEALTH IMPACT

Preventing Childhood Obesity: Health in the Balance, edited by Jeffrey P.
Koplan, Catharyn T. Liverman, and Vivica I. Kraak. Report of the Insti-
tute of Medicine of the National Academies. Published by the National
Academies Press, Washington, DC, 2005.

*The Surgeon General's Call to Action to Prevent and Decrease Overweight
and Obesity,* by the U.S. Department of Health and Human Services,

Public Health Service, Office of the Surgeon General, 2001. Available from the U.S. Government Printing Office (*http://www.surgeongeneral. gov/library*), Washington, DC.

http://www.cdc.gov/nccdphp/dnpa/bmi   This Centers for Disease Control and Prevention (CDC) Web site explains the significance of BMI as an indicator of weight status for adults, children, and adolescents. Users can input their height and weight into a "BMI Calculator" and follow a link to obtain the CDC's growth charts for babies, children, and adolescents.

HEALTHY EATING

Be Healthy! It's a Girl Thing: Food, Fitness, and Feeling Great, by Mavis Jukes and Lilian W. Y. Cheung. Published by Crown Books for Young Readers, New York, NY, 2003. An upbeat guide to improving nutrition, fitness, and self-image for girls in grades 5 to 9.

Child of Mine: Feeding with Love and Good Sense, by Ellyn Satter. Published by Bull Publishing Company, Boulder, CO, 2000. Satter is a registered dietitian whose readable, commonsense approach to feeding infants and children earns favorable recommendations from nutrition experts. Other books by her are also recommended.

Eat, Drink, and Be Healthy: The Harvard Medical School Guide to Healthy Eating, by Walter C. Willett, M.D., Ph.D. Published by Simon & Schuster, New York, NY, 2001. Epidemiologist Willett offers an alternative version of the Food Guide Pyramid with increased emphasis on dietary sources of "healthy" fats and whole grains. Includes recipes and menus.

American Academy of Pediatrics Guide to Your Child's Nutrition: Making Peace at the Table and Building Healthy Habits for Life, by William H. Dietz, M.D., Loraine Stern, M.D., and the American Academy of Pediatrics. Published by Villard, New York, NY, 1999. Information and strategies for feeding kids, from newborns to adolescents.

The Stoplight Diet for Children, by Leonard H. Epstein, Ph.D. and Sally Squires, M.S. Published by Little, Brown and Co., Boston, MA, 1988. (Out of print, but may be available from public libraries or used bookstores.) Forms the basis for eating plans and dietary counseling approaches used in many pediatric obesity treatment programs.

Volumetrics: Feel Full on Fewer Calories, by Barbara J. Rolls, Ph.D., and Robert A. Barnett. Published by HarperCollins, New York, NY, 2000. Based on research showing that eating nutritious foods that are low in energy density (such as fresh vegetables and fruits) helps people feel satiated and prevents excess weight gain.

The Way to Eat, by David L. Katz, M.D., M.P.H., and Maura Harrigan Gonzalez, M.S., R.D. Published by Sourcebooks, Inc., Naperville, IL, 2002. Particularly helpful on personal and family strategies for changing unhealthy eating habits.

http://kidnetic.com   An interactive Web site for children ages 9 to 12 and their parents that promotes healthy eating and active living. It's a project of the International Food Information Council Foundation (*http://www.ific.org*), whose Web site also offers general nutrition information and child-feeding tips for parents. IFIC is supported by the food, beverage, and agricultural industries.

http://www.cfsan.fda.gov/~dms/lab-gen.html   Learn how to read and interpret the nutrition information on food labels at this Web address, part of the Food and Drug Administration's Web site. Also provides a lesson kit on food labels for high school teachers.

http://www.shapeup.org   Web site of Shape Up America!, a nonprofit organization dedicated to helping people achieve and maintain a healthy weight.

http://www.usda.gov   This is the U.S. Department of Agriculture's Web site. By clicking on the Food and Nutrition link, you can find the latest edition of the government's dietary guidelines, standard serving sizes, the Food Guide Pyramid (including recommended servings for children of different ages), facts about the federal school lunch program, and other valuable information. There's also an Interactive Healthy Eating Index and Physical Activity Tool that allows the user to input personal information about diet and activity patterns and get an individualized assessment.

EATING DISORDERS

Policy Statement: Identifying and Treating Eating Disorders, by the American Academy of Pediatrics, Committee on Adolescence. *Pediatrics,* vol. 111, pp. 204–211, 2003. Available at *http://aappolicy. aappublications.org.* Guidance for health professionals on identifying and treating children with eating disorders.

http://www.nimh.nih.gov/publicat/eatingdisorders.cfm   The National Institute of Mental Health Web site offers information about anorexia nervosa, bulimia, and binge eating disorders, including research, treatment, and links to specialty organizations and advocacy groups.

BOOSTING PHYSICAL ACTIVITY, REDUCING SCREEN TIME

http://americaonthemove.org   A national initiative to promote physical activity, described in Chapter 5.

http://www.aahperd.org/naspe/template.cfm   The Web site of the National Association for Sport and Physical Education, particularly useful for parents of school-age children, coaches, and P.E. teachers.

http://www.presidentschallenge.org   Interactive Web site promoting physical activity, sponsored by the President's Council on Physical Fitness and Sports.

http://www.tvallowance.com   The electronic TV monitor used in Stanford researcher Tom Robinson's study on preventing obesity by reducing children's TV-watching time (see Chapter 5) can be purchased at this Web site.

http://www.tv-turnoff.org   Web site for TV-Turnoff Network, devoted to helping children and families reduce their viewing time.

PREGNANCY, BREASTFEEDING, INFANT FEEDING

American Academy of Pediatrics New Mother's Guide to Breastfeeding, edited by Joan Younger Meek, with Sherill Tippins. Published by Bantam Books, New York, NY, 2002.

The Best Start in Life, by David Barker. Published by Century, The Random House Group Limited, London, 2003. Describes how a woman's diet and nutritional status during pregnancy may affect her unborn child's future health.

Caring for Your Baby and Young Child, revised edition, by the American Academy of Pediatrics. Published by Bantam, New York, 2004. Child care from birth through age 5, including the feeding of infants and toddlers.

What to Expect When You're Expecting, by Heidi Murkoff, Arlene Eisenberg, and Sandee Hathaway. Published by Workman, New York, 2002. Provides a detailed and clearly organized guide to pregnancy.

A Woman's Guide to Breastfeeding, by the American Academy of Pediatrics. Available at *http://www.aap.org/family/brstguid.htm*. Provides general information for women planning to breastfeed.

The Womanly Art of Breastfeeding, 7th edition, revised, by La Leche League International. A comprehensive guide to breastfeeding, available at *www.lalecheleague.org*. The league's Web site also offers many other kinds of support for nursing mothers.

For advice on infant feeding, also see the *American Academy of Pediatrics Guide to Your Child's Nutrition* and Satter's *Child of Mine* and other books, listed under HEALTHY EATING.

SCHOOL HEALTH AND NUTRITION POLICIES

Eat Well & Keep Moving: An Interdisciplinary Curriculum for Teaching Upper Elementary School Nutrition and Physical Activity, by Lilian W. Y. Cheung, Steven L. Gortmaker, and Hank Dart. Published by Human Kinetics, Champaign, IL, 2001.

Guidelines for School Health Programs to Promote Lifelong Healthy Eating, Centers for Disease Control and Prevention. *Morbidity and Mortality Weekly Report*, Vol. 45, No. RR-9, pp. 1–33, June 14, 1996. Available from *http://www.cdc.gov/mmwr/preview/mmwrhtml/00042446.htm*. This report summarizes strategies for promoting healthy eating among school-age children and adolescents and provides nutrition education guidelines for a comprehensive school health program.

Planet Health: An Interdisciplinary Curriculum for Teaching Middle School Nutrition and Physical Activity, by Jill Carter, Jean Wiecha, Karen Peterson, and Steven L. Gortmaker. Published by Human Kinetics, Champaign, IL, 2001.

http://apps.nccd.cdc.gov/shi Web site of the School Health Index, a self-assessment and planning tool from the CDC that schools can use to improve policies on health and safety. Also useful for parents trying to strengthen school programs on food and physical activity.

HELPING AN OVERWEIGHT CHILD

Helping Your Overweight Child, by the NIDDK Weight-Control Information Network, July 2004. Online brochure with advice for parents and a list of additional resources. Made available by the International Food Information Council Foundation at *http://ific.org/publications/*

brochures/overweightkidbroch.cfm. The Weight-Control Information Network also has other publications as well as information about finding obesity treatment available through its Web site, *http://www.niddk.nih.gov/health/nutrit/win.htm,* or by mail at 1 WIN Way, Bethesda, MD 20892-3665. WIN's toll-free number is 1-877-946-4627.

Trim Kids: The Proven 12-Week Plan That Has Helped Thousands of Children Achieve a Healthier Weight, by Melinda S. Sothern, T. Kristian von Almen, and Heidi Schumacher. Published by Harper Collins, New York, 2001. The approach to treatment for overweight kids described in this book was developed from clinical research at Louisiana State University's Pennington Biomedical Research Center. (See Chapter 8 for more details.)

http://www.clinicaltrials.gov Parents and others can find federally funded research programs on the treatment of childhood obesity by consulting this NIH Web site.

http://www.obesity.org/subs/childhood/healthrisks.shtml This American Obesity Association Web site has a good section (with many useful links) on the health risks, diagnosis, and treatment of child obesity.

CRAFTING LAWS AND POLICIES TO FIGHT OBESITY

Food Politics: How the Food Industry Influences Nutrition and Health, by Marion Nestle. Published by the University of California Press, Berkeley, 2002. A fascinating look at how lobbying by the food and agriculture industries influences every aspect of government nutrition policy, from dietary guidelines to the school lunch program.

http://www.cdc.gov/nccdphp/dnpa/nutrition.htm Scroll down to State Legislative Information to access a database sponsored by the CDC that lists state legislative initiatives on nutrition and physical activity.

http://www.acfn.org Web site of the American Council for Fitness and Nutrition, a nonprofit organization formed in 2003 by a coalition of food and beverage companies, trade associations, and nutrition advocates to "work toward comprehensive and achievable solutions to the nation's obesity epidemic." Lists federal government initiatives and some workplace and community-level efforts, as well as programs sponsored by food and beverage companies. It's a starting point for learning about the food industry's response to the epidemic. (Many corporations also provide information about their positions and initiatives on their own Web sites.)

http://www.eatright.org Web site of the American Dietetic Association (the nation's largest organization of food and nutrition professionals), which has a section on Government Affairs with helpful information on food policy.

http://www.ncsl.org/programs/health/pp/healthpromo.cfm Database sponsored by the National Conference of State Legislatures for looking up state legislation on many health topics.

http://www.publichealthadvocacy.org Web site of the California Center for Public Health Advocacy. Provides examples of how California nutrition activists have pioneered the approach of using specific local data on children's obesity and diabetes risk as a lobbying tool to engage voters and to encourage local and state legislators to pass new laws on school food and other issues. Activists in other cities and states are beginning to adopt this approach.

http://www.thecommunityguide.org This Web site of a nonfederal community task force on preventive services provides information on the strength of the evidence supporting various strategies for improving nutrition and promoting activity.

LIMITING THE MARKETING OF
PRODUCTS TO CHILDREN

Consuming Kids: The Hostile Takeover of Childhood, by Susan Linn. Published by New Press, New York, NY, 2004. A highly critical look at how American companies market their products to children.

The Role of Media in Childhood Obesity, by the Kaiser Family Foundation, 2004. Available at *http://www.kff.org*. This nonprofit organization is known for its research on health policy issues.

http://www.ana.net Web site of the Association of National Advertisers, a trade organization of more than 300 companies that collectively spend more than $100 billion on marketing and advertising. On the ANA's homepage, there is a link to a "white paper" describing the industry's current self-regulation guidelines for food advertising (*http://www.narcpartners.org/narcwhitepaper.aspx*) and you can also find advertisers' positions on current legislative and regulatory issues.

http://www.asu.edu/educ/epsl/ceru.htm Web site of the Commercialism in Education Research Unit, directed by Alex Molnar, a professor of education policy at Arizona State University. The center does both research and advocacy; its Web site contains a roundup of news about efforts opposing commercialism in schools in various parts of the country.

http://www.commercialalert.org Web site of a nonprofit organization, cofounded by Ralph Nader, whose mission statement says it aims "to keep the commercial culture within its proper sphere, and to prevent it from exploiting children."

http://*www.commercialfreechildhood.org* The Web site of the Campaign for a Commerical-Free Childhood (CCFC), formerly known as Stop Commercial Exploitation of Children (SCEC). Run by Boston psychologist Susan Linn, whose book is listed above, CCFC describes itself as a national coalition of health care professionals, educators, advocacy groups, and parents dedicated to countering the harmful effects of marketing to children.

http://www.cspinet.org Web site of the Center for Science in the Public Interest, a nonprofit Washington-based lobbying and advocacy group, best known for its long-standing activism on the nutritional content and marketing of fast food. Provides information on nutrition issues and policy initiatives.

http://www.obligation.org Web site of an Alabama-based nonprofit organization dedicated to fighting unrestricted marketing to children, particularly on television and in schools (as on Channel One). Obligation's founder, Jim Metlock, received an award from the Alabama chapter of the American Academy of Pediatrics.

PROMOTING PHYSICAL ACTIVITY IN COMMUNITIES

http://www.activeliving.org Web site for the Active Living Network, a project partially funded by the nonprofit Robert Wood Johnson Foundation. It's described as a national coalition of leaders seeking to create environments that support physical activity.

http://www.cdc.gov/nccdphp/dnpa/aces.htm Web site for Centers for Disease Control and Prevention's Active Community Environments Initiative, with additional resources on walking and biking trails and physical activity promotion.

http://www.cdc.gov/nccdphp/dnpa/kidswalk/index.htm The KidsWalk-to-School program on the CDC's Web site features a downloadable presentation, lesson plans, and other information for organizing a community program to get children to walk or bike to school.

http://www.nhlbi.nih.gov/health/prof/heart/obesity/hrt_n_pk/ Web site of Hearts N' Parks, a national community-based program supported by the National Heart, Lung, and Blood Institute that provides activities, resources, and training to people involved in park and recreation programs.

http://www.walkable.org Walkable Communities, Inc., is a nonprofit corporation headed by Dan Burden (a longtime activist for bicycle and pedestrian facilities in communities). The Web site provides information, training, planning services, and other assistance for groups and organizations seeking to make their communities more walkable and bikeable.

http://www.walktoschool-usa.org   Web site offering a toolkit and other resources for establishing a Safe Routes to School Program in your neighborhood.

PROMOTING ACCESS TO FRESH FOODS

The New Farmers' Market, by Vance Corum, Marcie Rosenzweig, and Eric Gibson. Available from New World (*www.nwpub.net/nfm.html*), Auburn, CA, 2001. The Food Trust's Brian Lang recommends this book for anyone who wants to learn how to start a farmers market.

http://www.ams.usda.gov/farmersmarkets/   Web site of the Agricultural Marketing Service of the U.S. Department of Agriculture. Contains a list of farmers markets in every state, as well as information on obtaining federal funding or linking up with private organizations to establish or expand local farmers markets.

http://www.healthystores.org   Web site of the Healthy Stores Project (described in Chapter 9). Includes sample materials used to educate local consumers and promote healthy foods, as well as a list of helpful links.

http://www.thefoodtrust.org   Web site of the Food Trust, a Philadelphia-based nonprofit organization that operates farmers markets, promotes better nutrition in schools, and works to improve local availability of fresh foods. Helpful for anyone who wants to pursue such activities. The Food Trust and the Healthy Stores Project (listed above) are also cooperating to form a national network of people and organizations around the country working on the issue of access to healthy foods.

Notes

CHAPTER 1

p. 5　the prevalence of obesity in the United States: Ogden, C. L., et al. 2002. *JAMA* 288(14):1728-1732.

p. 5　**The epidemic has spread to preschool-age children, even toddlers:** Koplan, J. P., et al., eds. 2005. *Preventing Childhood Obesity: Health in the Balance.* Institute of Medicine. Washington, DC: The National Academies Press.

p. 6　Figure: **Trends in childhood obesity in U.S. girls and boys aged 6 through 19 years:** Ogden, C. L., M. D. Carroll, and C. L. Johnson. 2002. *JAMA* 288(14):1728-1732.

p. 6　**a majority of overweight kids and teenagers have already developed:** Freedman, D. S., et al. 1999. *Pediatrics* 103(6 Pt 1):1175-1182.

p. 7　**Julie Gerberding . . . declared obesity the number one health threat:** Reuters, October 28, 2003.

p. 12　**children represented by the "heavy" half of the curve . . . leaner children represented by the "light" half:** Flegal, K. M., and R. P. Troiano. 2000. *International Journal of Obesity* 24:807-818.

p. 12　Figure: **This schematic graph . . . helps illustrate the concept of**

BMI distribution shifts: Described in Flegal, K. M., and R. P. Troiano. 2000. *International Journal of Obesity* 24:807-818.

p. 14   **Among kids of both sexes ... 40 percent of Mexican Americans and 36 percent of African Americans:** Ogden, C. L., op cit.

p. 14   **The prevalence of obesity among 7-year-old American Indian children:** Caballero, B., et al. 2003. *American Journal of Clinical Nutrition* 78:308-312.

p. 15   **probably much more difficult to avoid ingesting too many calories:** Drewnowski, A., and S. E. Specter. 2004. *American Journal of Clinical Nutrition* 79:6-16.

p. 15   **placed the annual toll of obesity and inactivity at 400,000 deaths per year:** Mokdad, A. H., et al. 2004. *JAMA* 291(10):1238-1245. On November 23, 2004, as this book went to press, the *Wall Street Journal* reported that the CDC was conducting an internal review of computational errors made in this study and was expected to revise downward its estimate of the annual number of deaths linked to obesity. The article said that the study's authors planned to submit an erratum or correction to the *Journal of the American Medical Association* after the CDC's internal inquiry was completed.

p. 16   **Almost 80 percent of obese adults ... have one of those conditions:** Koplan, J. P., and W. H. Dietz.1999. *JAMA* 282:1579-1581.

p. 16   **cost of hospitalizations of children ... for obesity-related illnesses tripled:** Dietz, W. H. 2004. *New England Journal of Medicine* 350:855-857.

p. 16   **the incidence of this type of diabetes in children rose tenfold:** Pinhas-Hamiel, O., et al. 1996. *Journal of Pediatrics* 128:608-615.

p. 16   **Thirty percent of boys and 40 percent of girls ... will become diabetic:** Narayan, K. M., et al. 2003. *JAMA* 290:1884-1890.

p. 17   **Indeed, type 2 diabetes may be a more rapidly progressive disease in children than in adults:** Styne, D. M. 2001. *Pediatric Clinics of North America* 48(4):823-854.

p. 18   **Almost 30 percent of overweight children ... have the metabolic syndrome:** Cook, S., et al. 2003. *Archives of Pediatrics & Adolescent Medicine* 157:821-827.

p. 18   **a recent national study found that between 1988 and 2000 the average blood pressure of children in the United States edged upward by a couple of points:** Muntner, P., et al. 2004. *JAMA* 291:2107-2113.

p. 18   **Researchers have also documented worrisome changes in the hearts and arteries of obese children:** Woo, K. S., et al. 2004. *Circulation* 109:1981-1986.

p. 19   **About two-thirds of people who are overweight or obese as adults were not overweight during the first 20 years of their lives:** Bray, G. A. 2002. *American Journal of Clinical Nutrition* 76(3):497-498.

p. 19   "may be ideal candidates for treatment because the parents still have the opportunity to influence their children's activity and diet positively": Whitaker, R. C., et al. 1997. *New England Journal of Medicine* 337:869-873.

p. 20   classified as "lean" if their BMI fell between the 25th and 50th percentiles: Must, A., et al. 1992. *New England Journal of Medicine* 327:1350-1355.

p. 20   Recently a much larger study found that being overweight in adolescence affects adult mortality rates about equally in both sexes: Engeland, A., et al. 2003. *American Journal of Epidemiology* 157:517-523.

p. 21   being severely obese as a young adult reduces life expectancy more in black men than in white men: Fontaine, K. R., et al. 2003. *JAMA* 289(2):187-193.

p. 21   These findings . . . have been criticized on various technical grounds: Manson, J. E., and S. S. Bassuk. 2003. *JAMA* 289(2):229-230.

CHAPTER 2

p. 29   When the gene for leptin was identified and sequenced in 1994: Zhang, Y., et al. 1994. *Nature* 372:425-432.

p. 30   In little more than a decade, scientists have sketched the broad outlines of the biological system that regulates body weight: Sources for the scientific explanation that follows: Flier, J. S. 2004. *Cell* 116:337-350; Spiegelman, B. M., and J. S. Flier. 2001. *Cell* 104:531-543.

p. 32   The fall in leptin triggers: Leibel, R. L. 2002. *Nutrition Reviews* 60(10):S15-S19.

p. 34   when people are presented with appetizing, good-smelling food, many regions of the brain become metabolically active: Wang, G. L., et al. 2004. *Neuroimage* 21(4):1790-1797.

p. 34   The ubiquitous transmitter chemicals dopamine and serotonin . . . are also believed to affect feeding behavior and the rewarding aspects of food: Saper, C. B., et al. 2002. *Neuron* 36:199-211.

p. 35   Findings like these may help explain why people who are depressed or anxious often seek out specific "comfort foods": Dallman, M. F., et al. 2003. *Proceedings of the National Academy of Sciences of the United States of America* 100(20):11696-11701.

p. 35   fat cells actively metabolize steroid hormones such as male and female sex hormones: Kershaw, E. E., and J. S. Flier. 2004. *Journal of Clinical Endocrinology & Metabolism* 89(6):2548-2556.

p. 36   a team of British researchers led by Stephen O'Rahilly reported the cases of two children . . . who had suffered from severe obesity since infancy: Montague, C. T., et al. 1997. *Nature* 387:903-908.

p. 40   Stunkard concluded that hereditary factors account for about 70 percent of obesity and environmental factors for only about 30 percent: Stunkard, A. J., et al. 1990. *New England Journal of Medicine* 322:1483-1487.

p. 41   "Genetic influences have an important role in determining human fatness in adults," the research team concluded: Stunkard, A. J., et al. 1986. *New England Journal of Medicine* 314:193-198.

p. 41   researchers concluded that genes account for only about 25 to 40 percent of the variation in people's tendency to store excess body fat: Bouchard, C., et al. 2003. *Genetics of Human Obesity.* In: Bray, G. A., and C. Bouchard, eds. *Handbook of Obesity, Etiology and Pathophysiology.* Second Edition. New York: Marcel Dekker, Inc.

p. 41   Some researchers suggest that people can probably be categorized according to their degree of inherited risk ... and genetic resistance to becoming overweight: Loos, R. J., and C. Bouchard. 2003. *Journal of Internal Medicine* 254(5):401-425.

p. 42   research indicates that the influence of genetics on body weight is as strong as its influence on height: Flier, J. S. 2004. *Cell* 116:337-350.

p. 42   Studies of twins tell us that genetics plays as great a role in establishing obesity risk: Stunkard, A. J. 1986. *JAMA* 256:51-54.

p. 44   That's less than 1 percent of an adult's average daily intake: Weigle, D. S. 1994. *FASEB Journal* 8(3):302-310.

p. 47   They practiced traditional methods of agriculture and farming until white settlers diverted the Gila River: Tataranni, P. A. 2001. *Reviews in Endocrine & Metabolic Disorders* 2:365-369.

p. 48   In a 1994 study Ravussin compared a group of Arizona Pimas with a group of Pimas: Ravussin, E., et al. 1994. *Diabetes Care* 17:1067-1074.

p. 49   In a 2002 study Robert S. Lindsay and colleagues reported that the pattern of weight gain in Pima children differs markedly from U.S. national norms: Lindsay, R. S., et al. 2002. *Pediatrics* 109:e33. [Online]. Available at: http://www.pediatrics.org/cgi/content/full/109/2/e33 [accessed November 12, 2004].

p. 49   A 2002 study by Arline D. Salbe and colleagues found that Pima 5- and 10-year-olds who participated in more sports ... were less likely to be obese: Salbe, A. D., et al. 2002. *Pediatrics* 110:307-314.

CHAPTER 3

p. 56   In a survey by Stanford University researchers of more than 900 California third-grade students: Robinson, T. N., et al. 2001. *Journal of Pediatrics* 138:181-187.

p. 56   **Among white girls, higher socioeconomic status and higher levels of education are associated with lower levels of obesity:** Kimm, S. Y., et al. 1996. *Annals of Epidemiology* 6:266-275.

p. 58   **Its relative frequency in other racial or ethnic groups is uncertain:** [Online]. Available at: http://www.nimh.nih.gov/publicat/eating disorders.cfm [accessed November 9, 2004].

p. 60   **A majority did not routinely perform recommended checks . . . all serious problems that can develop in obese kids:** Barlow, S. E., et al. 2002. *Pediatrics* 110:222-228.

p. 61   **somewhat more realistic about their own body size:** Baughcum, A. E., et al. 2000. *Pediatrics* 106:1380-1386.

p. 61   **Making parents aware of the health risks for children of being overweight:** American Academy of Pediatrics Committee on Nutrition. 2003. *Pediatrics* 112:424-430.

p. 62   **At least one state—Arkansas—is in the process of adopting such a program statewide:** Judith Graham, "Arkansas to grade kids on obesity." Chicago Tribune. September 15, 2003.

p. 62   **Among parents of overweight kids who did not receive such reports:** Chomitz, V. R., et al. 2003. *Archives of Pediatrics & Adolescent Medicine* 157:765-772.

p. 63   **girls and boys who were frequent dieters gained more weight annually than those who never dieted:** Field, A. E., et al. 2003. *Pediatrics* 112:900-906.

p. 63   **"They hate the fact that Briana is heavy and try to pin it on me":** Balancing Act, by Sherry Arria as told to Liz Welch, New York Times Magazine. September 7, 2003.

p. 64   **Johnson and Birch found that the very children whose mothers tried hardest to control how much they ate:** Johnson, S. L., and L. L. Birch. 1994. *Pediatrics* 94(5):653-661.

p. 64   **Girls who had been overweight at 5 . . . showed the greatest degree of overeating at the age of 9:** Birch, L. L., et al. 2003. *American Journal of Clinical Nutrition* 78(2):215-220.

p. 65   **early dietary restriction may predispose girls:** Birch, L. L., and J. O. Fisher. 1998. *Pediatrics* 101:539-549.

p. 65   **concluded that girls whose parents controlled their food intake tended to be less overweight, not more so:** Robinson, T. N., et al. 2001. *Obesity Research* 9(5):306-312.

p. 67   **stigmatization of overweight children has worsened in recent decades:** Latner, J. D., and A. J. Stunkard. 2003. *Obesity Research* March 11(3):452-456.

p. 67   **One study found that overweight girls . . . were less likely to gain acceptance to elite colleges than their slender peers:** Canning, H., and J. Mayer. 1966. *New England Journal of Medicine* 275:1172-1174.

p. 67   the National Longitudinal Survey of Youth, found that women who were obese in late adolescence and young adulthood: Gortmaker, S. L., et al. 1993. *New England Journal of Medicine* 329:1008-1012.

p. 68   girls who expressed concern about their weight: Erickson, S. J., et al. 2000. *Archives of Pediatrics & Adolescent Medicine* 154(9):931-935.

p. 68   Robinson found, body size . . . was the strongest predictor of body dissatisfaction: Robinson, T. N., et al. 1996. *Journal of Adolescent Health* December 19(6):384-393.

p. 68   those who were very overweight did have more negative feelings about their appearance: Young-Hyman, D., et al. 2003. *Journal of Pediatric Psychology* 28(7):463-472.

p. 69   two to three times more likely to consider or attempt suicide than those who had not: Eisenberg, M. E., et al. 2003. *Archives of Pediatrics & Adolescent Medicine* 157:733-738.

p. 69   Overweight children were almost twice as likely as lean children not to be named as a friend: Strauss, R. S., and H. A. Pollack. 2003. *Archives of Pediatrics & Adolescent Medicine* 157:746-752.

p. 70   "I don't have to conform to your images": Courtesy of Michael Rich. From a collection of video clips viewed at Children's Hospital, Boston, on June 3, 2003.

p. 70   Researchers Elizabeth Goodman and Robert C. Whitaker performed a prospective study of more than 9,000 children: Goodman, E., and R. C. Whitaker. 2002. *Pediatrics* 110(3):497-504.

CHAPTER 4

p. 82   "It is not likely that we will ever return the environment": Hill, J. O., et al. 2003. *Science* 299(5608):853-855.

p. 82   The amount of food available to the U.S. population: French, S. A., et al. 2001. *Annual Review of Public Health* 22:309-335.

p. 82   average daily caloric intake for women in 1999–2000: McKay, B. Wall Street Journal. February 6, 2004.

p. 83   the NHANES have consistently documented: Centers for Disease Control and Prevention. 2004. *MMWR* 53:80-82.

p. 83   these cross-sectional studies—"snapshots" of dietary intake at different points in time: Wright, J. D., et al. 2003. Advance Data from Vital and Health Statistics April 17(334):1-4; Gleason, P., and C. Suitor. 2001. United States Department of Agriculture, Food and Nutrition Service Report No. CN-01-CD1; Nielsen, S. J., et al. 2002. *Obesity Research* 10:370-378; Morton, J. F., and J. F. Guthrie. 1998. *Family Economics and Nutrition Review* 11:44-57.

p. 83   **Americans reduced their fat intake between 1970 and 1994:**
French, S. A., et al. 2001. *Annual Review of Public Health* 22:309-335.

p. 83   **One analysis of children's intake:** Morton, J. F., and J. F. Guthrie,
op cit.

p. 84   **Milk consumption decreased by 37 percent in adolescent boys:**
Cavandini, C., et al. 2000. *Archives of Disease in Childhood* 83:18-24.

p. 84   **one-third of girls and more than half of boys are drinking
three or more . . . soft drinks per day:** Guthrie, J. F., and J. F. Morton. 2000.
Journal of the American Dietetic Association 100:43-51.

p. 84   **currently make up 16 percent of Americans' total calorie intake:** French, S. A., et al., op cit.

p. 84   **linked soft drink consumption with higher total daily calorie
intake and increased risk of obesity:** Ludwig, D. S., et al. 2001. *Lancet*
357:505-508.

p. 85   **The same study also showed that high intake of sugar-sweetened soft drinks or fruit punch:** Schulze, M. B., et al. 2004. *JAMA* 292:927-
934.

p. 85   **In 1996 Americans ate an average of 1.3 servings of fruit per
day:** French, S. A., et al., op cit.

p. 85   **children ate an average of 4.1 servings of fruits and vegetables
daily:** Gleason, P., and C. Suitor, op cit.

p. 86   **dark green and orange vegetables . . . made up only 8 percent of
kids' vegetable intake:** Centers for Disease Control. *National Health and Nutrition Examination Survey, National Center for Health Statistics.* [Online].
Available at: http://www.cdc.gov/nchs/ppt/hpdata2010/focusareas/
fa19.ppt#16 [accessed November 12, 2004].

p. 86   **five vegetables—iceberg lettuce, frozen potatoes, fresh potatoes, potato chips, and canned tomatoes:** Putnam, J., et al. 2002. *Food Review* 25:2-15.

p. 86   **In 1997 nearly half of family expenditures for food were spent
on food and drink prepared outside the home:** Putnam, J., et al. 1999. Pp.
133-160 in: Frazao, E., ed. *America's Eating Habits: Changes and Consequences.* Washington, DC: Economic Research Service, United States Department of Agriculture; Agriculture Information Bulletin No. 750.

p. 86   **consumption of foods prepared away from home made up almost a third of children's total calorie intake:** Lin, B. H., et al. 1999. Pp.
213-242 in: Frazao, E., ed. *America's Eating Habits: Changes and Consequences.* Washington, DC: Economic Research Service, United States Department of Agriculture; Agriculture Information Bulletin No. 750.

p. 86   **Although all the kids in the study tended to overconsume fast
food:** Ebbeling, C. B., et al. 2004. *JAMA* 291(23):2828-2833.

p. 87   The recent expansion in the nation's portion sizes started as a marketing strategy: Nielsen, S. J., and B. M. Popkin. 2003. *JAMA* 289:450-453.

p. 87   Today, a regular can of Coca-Cola holds 12 ounces: Pendergrast, M. 2000. *For God, Country, and Coca Cola: The Definitive History of the Great American Soft Drink and the Company That Makes It.* New York: Basic Books.

p. 87   The ballooning of portion sizes is reflected on grocery store shelves and even in cookbook recipes: Young, L. R., and M. Nestle. 2002. *American Journal of Public Health* 92:246-249.

p. 88   as children grow older, they become responsive to environmental cues: Rolls, B. J., et al. 2000. *Journal of the American Dietetic Association* 100:232-234.

p. 88   Rolls and colleagues found that when they doubled the size of an entree served at lunch: Fisher, J. O., B. J. Rolls, and L. L. Birch. 2003. *American Journal of Clinical Nutrition* 77:1164-1170.

p. 88   Food manufacturers, retailers, and services are second only to the automobile industry: Gallo, A. E. 1999. In: Frazao, E., ed. *America's Eating Habits: Changes and Consequences.* Washington, DC: Economic Research Service, United States Department of Agriculture; Agriculture Information Bulletin No. 750.

p. 88   Food and beverage advertisers spend an estimated: Nestle, M. 2002. *Food Politics: How the Food Industry Influences Nutrition and Health.* Berkeley, CA: University of California Press. P. 179.

p. 88   One study found that television commercials influence: Borzekowski, D. L., and T. N. Robinson. 2001. *Journal of the American Dietetic Association* 101:42-46.

p. 88   McDonald's spent almost $572 million: French, S. A., et al. 2001. *Annual Review of Public Health* 22:309-335.

p. 89   Hill writes, "as a society, we should be more willing ... to carefully manage the food and physical activity environments": Hill, J. O., et al. 2003. *Science* 299:853-855.

p. 90   Recent studies in children and adults have also found that those who eat breakfast regularly: Albertson, A. M., et al. 2003. *Journal of the American Dietetic Association* 103:1613-1619; Pereira, M. A. Report at American Heart Association meeting. March 6, 2003.

p. 90   It also appears that there is nothing magic about a three-meals-a-day schedule: Yunsheng, M., et al. 2003. *American Journal of Epidemiology* 158(1):85-92.

p. 91   found that those who ate dinner at home with their families consumed fewer fried foods: Gillman, M. W., et al. 2000. *Archives of Family Medicine* 9:235-240.

pp. 92-93   those who were taught to focus on noticing the sensation of fullness in their stomachs: Birch, L. L., et al. 1987. *Learning and Motivation* 18:301-317.

p. 93   research has shown that even picky toddlers eat an appropriate and consistent number of calories: Birch, L. L., et al. 1991. *New England Journal of Medicine* 324:232-235.

p. 95   When the USDA's familiar Food Guide Pyramid . . . was first released in 1992: Willett, W. C., and M. J. Stampfer. 2003. *Scientific American* January:64-71.

p. 96   During the same period, an increasing proportion of the population has become overweight or obese: Willett, W. C. 2001. *Eat, Drink, and Be Healthy: The Harvard Medical School Guide to Healthy Eating.* New York: Simon & Schuster. P. 45.

p. 96   It also notes the evidence linking sugar-sweetened beverages and weight gain: 2005 Report of the Dietary Guidelines Advisory Committee. [Online]. Available at: http://www.health.gov/dietaryguidelines/dga2005/report [accessed November 11, 2004].

p. 99   Table: **Types of Dietary Fat:** reprinted with the permission of Simon & Schuster Adult Publishing Group from *Eat, Drink, and Be Healthy: The Harvard Medical School Guide to Healthy Eating* by Walter C. Willett, M.D. Copyright © 2001 by President and Fellows of Harvard College.

p. 100   An authoritative report on dietary intake was issued in 2002 by the Institute of Medicine: Institute of Medicine. 2002. *Dietary Reference Intakes for Energy, Carbohydrate, Fiber, Fat, Fatty Acids, Cholesterol, Protein, and Amino Acids (Macronutrients).* Washington, DC: The National Academies Press.

p. 101   Examples of items to be removed from kitchen shelves . . . might be fried chips, candy, and high-fat baked goods: Katz, D. L. 2002. *The Way to Eat.* Naperville, IL: Sourcebooks, Inc.

p. 103   urges that large clinical trials be carried out in overweight adults: Parikh, S. J., and J. A. Yanovski. 2003. *American Journal of Clinical Nutrition* 77:281-287.

p. 104   People who regularly eat lots of fruits and vegetables: Willett, W. C., op cit.

p. 104   Vegetables with a hard surface: Food Safety and Inspection Service, USDA. Does Washing Food Promote Food Safety? [Online]. Available at: http://www.fsis.usda.gov/OA/pubs/washing.htm [accessed November, 11, 2004].

p. 105   researchers found that a diet containing 8 to 10 servings of fruits and vegetables per day: Moore, T., et al. 2001. *The DASH Diet for Hypertension.* New York: Simon & Schuster.

p. 105   Some fiber remains solid (insoluble) in the digestive tract: Willett, W. C., op cit.

p. 106   **The site has a helpful chart of serving sizes:** [Online]. Available at: http://www.health.gov/dietaryguidelines/ [accessed November 11, 2004].

p. 107   **Rolls's findings form the basis for a practical, relatively low-fat approach to eating:** Rolls, B. J., and R. A. Barnett. 2000. *Volumetrics.* New York: HarperCollins.

p. 107   **some experts recommend dividing each person's dinner plate into imaginary sections:** American Institute for Cancer Research. The New American Plate. [Online]. Available at: www.aicr.org/publications/nap/nap2.lasso [accessed November 11, 2004].

p. 107   **It's a good idea to keep plenty of "green" foods visible:** Epstein, L. H., and S. Squires. 1988. *The Stoplight Diet for Children.* Boston: Little, Brown and Co.

p. 108   **contained the surprising finding that eating a potato raised blood glucose levels as rapidly:** Bantle, J. P., et al. 1983. *New England Journal of Medicine* 309:7-12.

p. 108   **found that low-glycemic-index diets improve blood sugar control in diabetes:** Ludwig, D. S. 2002. *JAMA* 287:2414-2423.

p. 109   **The third test meal had exactly the same number of calories as the other two:** Ludwig, D. S., et al. 1999. *Pediatrics* 103:E26.

p. 110   **those in the low-glycemic-index group . . . had lost significantly more weight and more fat:** Ebbeling, C. B., et al. 2003. *Archives of Pediatrics & Adolescent Medicine* 157:773-779.

p. 111   **"Increase consumption of fruits, vegetables and legumes":** Ludwig, D. S. 2002. *JAMA* 287:2414-2423.

CHAPTER 5

p. 119   **Texas, for example, recently legislated 135 minutes of activity a week:** Reinhart, D. "Schools learn how to get in more exercise time." Beaumont Enterprise. October 24, 2003.

p. 120   **The most highly educated Americans were the group most likely to engage in regular vigorous activity:** Barnes, P. M., and C. A. Schoenborn. 2003. *Advance Data from Vital and Health Statistics* May 14(333):1-23.

p. 121   **About one-quarter of participants said they did no moderate physical activity:** Spors, K. K. Wall Street Journal. October 21, 2003.

p. 121   **The step counts for girls were lower than for boys:** Vincent, S. D., et al. 2003. *Medicine and Science in Sports and Exercise* August 35(8):1367-1373.

p. 121   **A 1996 report of the U.S. Surgeon General recommends:**

Physical Activity and Health: A Report from the Surgeon General. 1996. Atlanta, GA: United States Department of Health and Human Services.

p. 122   **The Institute of Medicine recommends at least an hour of moderately intense activity daily:** Institute of Medicine. 2002. *Dietary Reference Intakes for Energy, Carbohydrate, Fiber, Fat, Fatty Acids, Cholesterol, Protein, and Amino Acids.* Washington, DC: The National Academies Press.

p. 122   **Concerns about traffic danger prevent an estimated 20 million children:** Centers for Disease Control and Prevention. 2002. *MMWR.* August 16;51(32):701-704.

p. 122   **Most children in grades 1 through 6 are enrolled in physical education:** Kohl, H. W., and K. E. Hobbs. 1998. *Pediatrics* 101:549-554.

p. 122   **students engaged in only about three minutes of moderate to vigorous exercise:** Sallis, J. F., et al. 1997. *American Journal of Public Health* 87:1328-1334.

p. 122   **children may average as little as 10 minutes per week of moderate to vigorous activity in school P.E. classes:** Robinson, T. N. 2001. Pp. 129-141 in: Johnston, F. E., and G. D. Foster, eds. *Obesity, Growth and Development.* London: Smith-Gordon and Company.

p. 122   **Fields and courts are so crowded:** Di Massa, C. M. "Campus Crowding Can Make PE a Challenge." Los Angeles Times. November 19, 2003.

p. 123   Figure: **The percentage of trips during normal school travel hours:** Special Report 269: The Relative Risks of School Travel. 2002. Washington, DC: Transportation Research Board, National Research Council. P. 88.

p. 123   **About half of U.S. schools require physical education for students in grades 1 through 5:** Burgeson, C. R., et al. 2001. *Journal of School Health* 71:279-293.

p. 123   **Higher family incomes . . . linked to higher physical activity levels:** Gordon-Larsen, P., et al. 2000. *Pediatrics* 105(6):e83.

p. 123   **Along with declining overall activity levels:** Aaron, D. J., et al. 2002. *Archives of Pediatrics & Adolescent Medicine* 156:1075-1080.

p. 124   **activity levels fall by 64 percent for white girls and by 100 percent for black girls:** Kimm, S. Y., et al. 2002. *New England Journal of Medicine* 347(10):709-715.

p. 124   **About half of high school girls report:** Goran, M. I., et al. 1999. *International Journal of Obesity* 23(Suppl 3):S18-S33.

p. 125   **boys also retain fairly constant levels of aerobic power relative to their body mass:** Kohl, H. W., op cit.

p. 125   **The girls' food intake (adjusted for their weight):** Goran, M. I., et al. 1998. *Pediatrics* 101(5):887-891.

p. 126 **The body fat content of children in the program:** Luepker, R. V., et al. 1998. *Journal of Nutritional Biochemistry* 9:525-534.

p. 126 **The federally sponsored program Pathways:** Caballero, B., et al. 2003. *American Journal of Clinical Nutrition* 78:1030-1038.

p. 127 **But SPARK participants did not increase their activity levels outside school:** Sallis, J. F., et al. 1997. *American Journal of Public Health* 87(8):1328-1334.

p. 127 **those in the endurance group were not only fitter but showed a significant reduction in fatness:** Dwyer, T., et al. 1983. *International Journal of Epidemiology* 12:308-313.

p. 128 **girls in the Dance for Health classes significantly lowered their BMIs and their resting heart rates:** Flores, R. 1995. *Public Health Report* March-April;110(2):189-193.

p. 133 **Robinson estimated that . . . children in the United States spend an average of more than three years of their waking lives watching TV:** Robinson, T. N. 1998. *JAMA* 279:959-960.

p. 133 **One-quarter of children in this age group have a television in their bedrooms:** Henry J. Kaiser Family Foundation. Fall 2003. *Zero to Six: Electronic Media in the Lives of Infants, Toddlers and Preschoolers.* [Online]. Available at: http://www.kff.org/entmedia/3378.cfm [accessed November 12, 2004].

p. 133 **the average time spent in such pursuits rises to 4.5 hours per day:** Robinson, T. N. 2001. *Pediatric Clinics of North America* 48(4):1017-1025.

p. 134 Figure: **Daily media use among children:** Kids & Media @ The New Millennium, #1535, Henry J. Kaiser Family Foundation. November 1999. This information was reprinted with permission of the Henry J. Kaiser Family Foundation. The Foundation, based in Menlo Park, California, is a non-profit, independent national health care philanthropy and is not associated with Kaiser Permanente or Kaiser Industries.

p. 134 **Gortmaker suggested that a "dose-response relationship" exists:** Gortmaker, S. L., et al. 1996. *Archives of Pediatrics & Adolescent Medicine* 150:356-362.

p. 134 **evidence indicating that TV watching was a contributing factor to weight gain:** Dietz, W. H., and S. L. Gortmaker. 1985. *Pediatrics* 75:807-812.

p. 134 **preschoolers with a TV set in their bedrooms:** Dennison, B. A., et al. 2002. *Pediatrics* 109:1028-1035.

p. 135 **Food and drink consumed while watching television:** Matheson, D. M., et al. 2004. *American Journal of Clinical Nutrition* 79:1088-1094.

p. 135 **children younger than 7 or 8 do not understand that com-**

mercials are different from other program content: Wilcox, B. L., et al. 2004. Report of the APA Task Force on Advertising and Children. Washington DC: American Psychological Association.

p. 136   A 2001 study found that in families that watched television during two or more meals per day: Coon, K. A., et al. 2001. *Pediatrics* 107:e7.

p. 136   A recent Australian study found that people who eat lying down: Mundell, E. J. Reuters Health. Report on an oral presentation by Deirdre O'Donovan of the University of Adelaide at the Digestive Disease Week conference in Orlando, Florida. May 20, 2003.

p. 136   watching TV may consume even less energy than other sedentary activities: Klesges, R. C., et al. 1993. *Pediatrics* 91:281-286.

p. 136   Television watching was among the sedentary activities targeted: Epstein, L. H., et al. 1995. *Journal of Health Psychology* 14:109-115.

p. 137   Children in the schools where Planet Health was introduced: Gortmaker, S. L., et al. 1999. *Archives of Pediatrics & Adolescent Medicine* 153:409-418.

p. 137   Girls and overweight boys in the study who increased their physical activity level: Berkey, C. S., et al. 2003. *Pediatrics.* 111:836-843.

p. 137   Children's TV and video time should be limited: Dietz, W. H., and S. L. Gortmaker. 1993. *Pediatrics* 91:499-501.

p. 138   "Take note of the times when you watch TV but aren't really interested": Carter, J., J. Wiecha, K. Peterson, and S. L. Gortmaker. 2001. *Planet Health: An Interdisciplinary Curriculum for Teaching Middle School Nutrition and Physical Activity.* Champaign, IL: Human Kinetics Publishing. P. 30.

p. 141   The authors speculated that the daily walking done by the city-dwellers made the difference: Ewing, R., et al. 2003. *American Journal of Health Promotion* 18(1):47-57.

p. 142   Kids whose parents are physically active are almost six times as likely: Moore, L. L., et al. 1991. *Journal of Pediatrics* 118:215-219.

p. 142   At least one study suggests that parental activity levels are more closely correlated: Gottlieb, N. H., and M. S. Chen.1985. *Social Science & Medicine* 21:533-539.

p. 143   Experiences likely to prejudice children against continuing to participate in sports: American Academy of Pediatrics, Committee on Sports Medicine and Fitness and Committee on School Health. 2001. *Pediatrics* 107:1459-1462.

p. 147   Its national parent program, America on the Move, is sponsored primarily by food and beverage companies: [Online]. Available at: http://www.ppheal.org/our_sponsors.html [accessed November 12, 2004].

CHAPTER 6

p. 152   **the environment in the womb can affect an individual's later risk of obesity:** Oken, E., and M. W. Gillman. 2003. *Obesity Research* 11:496-506.

p. 153   **the rates of obesity and overweight grew faster among women of childbearing age:** Cogswell, M. E., et al. 2001. *Primary Care Update for Ob/Gyns* 8:89-105.

p. 153   **The percentage of pregnant women who gain more than 40 pounds during their pregnancies has been rising:** Martin, J. A., et al. 2003. Births: Final Data for 2002. Centers for Disease Control and Prevention. National Vital Statistics Reports 52:1-114.

p. 154   **They have a higher frequency of stillbirth than women who are not overweight:** Sebire, N. J., et al. 2001. *International Journal of Obesity* 25:1175-1182.

p. 154   **Their babies also have higher rates of several types of birth defects:** Watkins, M. L., et al. 2003. *Pediatrics* 111:1152-1158.

p. 154   **the percentage of pregnant women who fail to gain even this minimum amount:** Martin, J. A., et al., op cit.

p. 155   **Full-term infants are considered appropriate for gestational age:** Medline Plus: Medical Encyclopedia. [Online]. Available at: http://www.nlm.nih.gov/medlineplus/ [accessed November 12, 2004].

p. 157   **Infants of diabetic mothers "are born large but decrease their weight into a normal range":** Styne, D. M. 2001. *Pediatric Clinics of North America* 48:823-854.

p. 157   **Researchers at Northwestern University monitored children of diabetic mothers:** Silverman, B. L., et al. 1995. *Diabetes Care* 18:611-617.

p. 158   **researchers found that those who had been exposed to diabetes before birth had a higher frequency of obesity:** Dabelea, D., et al. 2000. *Diabetes* 49:2208-2211.

p. 158   **Almost all have found a direct association: "Higher birth weight is associated with higher attained BMI":** Oken, E., and M. W. Gillman, op cit.

p. 159   **the association between high birth weight and later obesity risk was reduced but not eliminated:** Gillman, M. W., et al. 2003. *Pediatrics* 111(3):e221-e226.

p. 160   **newborn rats fed a high-carbohydrate diet respond by producing excessive amounts of insulin even as adults and become obese:** Aalinkeel, R., et al. 2001. *American Journal of Physiology-Endocrinology and Metabolism* 281:E640-E648.

p. 160   **The leptin surge had to occur during a critical period in early life:** Bouret, S. G., et al. 2004. *Science* 304:108-110.

p. 160 **"Nutritional or other environmental factors that suppress leptin during brain development":** Oregon Health & Science University, press release. April 1, 2004.

p. 160 **In rats that were "overfed" from birth by being raised in unusually small litters:** Davidowa, H., et al. 2002. *NeuroReport* 13:1523-1527; Li, Y., et al. 2002. *Neuroscience Letters* 330:33-36.

p. 162 **certain aspects of the Dutch study's design may have reduced the validity of its findings:** Ravelli, G. P., et al. 1976. *New England Journal of Medicine* 295:349-353.

p. 162 **although two infants may be born with identical birth weights:** Barker, D. 2003. *The Best Start in Life.* London: Century. Pp. 52-53.

p. 163 **The mean birth weight for a "singleton" baby:** Martin, J. A., op cit.

p. 164 **Researchers do not have enough evidence yet to know whether some infants who are part of multiple births face similar health risks:** Barker, D., op cit., p. 79.

p. 165 **Despite the fact that almost half of nonpregnant women in the United States report that are they're trying to lose weight:** Cogswell, M. E., op cit.

p. 166 **adequate weight gain during pregnancy is very important for fetal growth:** Institute of Medicine: Committee on Nutritional Status During Pregnancy and Lactation, Food and Nutrition Board. 1990. *Nutrition During Pregnancy. Part 1, Weight Gain; Part II, Nutrient Supplements.* Washington, DC: National Academy Press.

p. 167 **Breastfeeding has many proven advantages over formula feeding:** American Academy of Pediatrics: Work Group on Breastfeeding. 1997. *Pediatrics* 100:1035-1039.

p. 168 **Despite the AAP's recommendations:** Li, R., et al. 2003. *Pediatrics* 111(5):1198-1201.

p. 169 **overweight women in general have more difficulty breastfeeding than slender women:** Li, R., et al. 2003. *American Journal of Clinical Nutrition* 77:931-936.

p. 169 **Only four studies suggested that breastfeeding provided some protection:** Butte, N. F., 2001. *Pediatric Clinics of North America* 48(1)189-198.

p. 170 **Kathryn G. Dewey ... recently assessed a group of larger and newer studies:** Dewey, K. G. 2003. *Journal of Human Lactation* 19:9-18.

p. 171 **rapid weight gain during the first four months of life was associated with a higher risk of being overweight at the age of 7:** Stettler, N., et al. 2002. *Pediatrics* 109(2):194-199.

p. 171 **showed that rapid weight gain in the early months of infancy was associated with a doubling of obesity risk at age 20:** Stettler, N., et al. 2003. *American Journal of Clinical Nutrition* 77:1374-1378.

p. 172   hopeful that future data from the PROBIT trial may help answer the question of whether breastfeeding really helps protect against later obesity: Kramer, M. S., et al. 2001. *JAMA* 285(4):413-420.

p. 173   Breastfed infants under 6 months old generally do not need water, juice, or other foods: American Academy of Pediatrics: Work Group on Breastfeeding. 1997. *Pediatrics* 100:1035-1039.

p. 175   Smell's key contribution to our perception of flavors explains why foods taste flat to us when we have a cold: Mennella, J. A. 1999. Pp. 104-113 in: Swaiman, K. F., and S. Ashwal, eds. *Pediatric Neurology*. St. Louis: Mosby, Inc.

p. 176   Animal research suggests that foods to which a fetus is exposed in this way may be preferred by the infant after birth: Mennella, J. A., op cit.

p. 176   showed that breast-fed infants stayed attached to the nipple longer: Mennella, J. A., and G. K. Beauchamp. 1993. *Pediatric Research* 34:805-808; Mennella, J. A., and G. K. Beauchamp, 1996. *Infant Behavior & Development* 19:13-19.

p. 176   Those who had been exposed to the flavor of carrot juice either before birth: Mennella, J. A., et al. 2001. *Pediatrics* 107:e88.

p. 177   A study by another pair of researchers found that breast-fed babies more readily accepted a new vegetable than did formula-fed ones: Sullivan, S. A., and L. L. Birch. 1994. *Pediatrics* 93:271-277.

p. 178   Such antibodies may be involved in causing damage to these insulin-producing cells: Ziegler, A. G., et al. 2003. *JAMA* 290:1721-1728; Norris, J. M., et al. 2003. *JAMA* 290:1713-1720.

p. 178   There was no statistically significant difference in sleep patterns or sleep duration: Macknin, M.L., et al. 1989. *American Journal of Diseases of Children* 143:1066-1068.

p. 179   (If a mother decides to stop breastfeeding before her infant is 6 months old, the baby should receive only formula until the age of 6 months.): American Academy of Pediatrics: Work Group on Breastfeeding. 1997. *Pediatrics* 100(6):1035-1039.

p. 179   "because ingesting new substances is a risky business, most new foods are not immediately accepted": Birch, L. L. 1998. *Journal of Nutrition* 128:407S-410S.

p. 179   preschool-age children who initially disliked certain vegetables began eating them after they saw other children eat them: Birch, L. L., and J. O. Fisher. 1998. *Pediatrics* 101:539-549.

p. 180   Although children in the study initially liked the lower-calorie and higher-calorie soups and yogurts equally well: Johnson, S. L., et al. 1991. *Physiology & Behavior* 50:1245-1251.

p. 180   It's unclear whether these children's preference was genetically based or whether it was influenced by exposure to high-fat foods in the home: Birch, L. L. 1998. *Journal of Nutrition.* 128:407S-410S.

p. 182   the emphasis is on training the appetite and teaching children to learn to eat the foods that adults eat: Stearns, P. N. 1997. *Fat History: Bodies and Beauty in the Modern World.* New York: New York University Press.

CHAPTER 7

p. 186   children who are involved in growing food in school gardens have been shown to increase their liking for certain vegetables: Morris, J., and S. Zidenberg-Cherr. 2002. *Journal of the American Dietetic Association* 102:91-93.

p. 191   detailed guidelines were published by the federal Centers for Disease Control and Prevention in 1996: Centers for Disease Control and Prevention. 1996. Guidelines for School Health Programs to Promote Lifelong Healthy Eating. *MMWR* June 14;45(RR-9):1-33.

p. 193   most school lunches contain a higher percentage of fat than the maximum specified by government requirements: General Accounting Office, School Lunch Program, May 2003. GAO-03-506.

p. 193   It is extremely rare for a school to lose its eligibility to participate in the federal school lunch program: Interview with Suanne Buggy, USDA public information officer, August 2004.

p. 193   Researcher Robert Whitaker found that about 30 percent of elementary school students spontaneously chose lower-fat menu items: Whitaker, R. C., et al. 1994. *Journal of Pediatrics* Oct;125(4):535-540.

p. 194   students who had learned about them in class ate from 3 to 20 times more of them than did the students in the control group: Demas, A. 1998. *American Journal of Cardiology* 82:80T-82T.

p. 194   And students were no longer allowed seconds at meals except for fruits and vegetables: Quad City Times, Gannett News Service. March 24, 2003.

p. 194   The USDA conducted a successful pilot program in several states: Buzby, J. C., et al. May 2003. Evaluation of the USDA Fruit and Vegetable Pilot Program. Report to Congress. USDA Economic Research Service. [Online]. Available at: http://www.fns.usda.gov/cnd/Research/FV030063.pdf [accessed November 12, 2004].

p. 195   found to her astonishment that they offered a total of 363 different snack and beverage items for sale: Statement of Vivian B. Pilant, South Carolina Department of Education, June 16, 2003, at Institute of Medicine workshop in Washington, DC.

p. 195   **Still, students often do have healthier alternatives:** Wechsler, H., et al. 2001. *Journal of School Health* 71:313-324.

p. 196   **"It wasn't something I relished doing, but we had to for our financial survival, plain and simple":** Lee, E. "Fast-food profits tempt schools." The Atlanta Journal-Constitution. May 5, 2003.

p. 196   **Machines dispensing soft drinks and fruit drinks are featured in the majority of U.S. schools:** General Accounting Office, op cit.

p. 196   **One Florida county school board agreed in 2000 to a five-year agreement with Pepsi-Cola worth $13.5 million:** Kerr, J. L. "Soft drink sales in schools face increasing criticism." The Florida Times-Union. March 16, 2004.

p. 196   **when prices for fresh fruit and baby carrots in a high school cafeteria were cut in half, sales of those items increased twofold to four-fold:** French, S. A., et al. 1997. *Journal of the American Dietetic Association* 97:1008-1010.

p. 196   **Since total sales from each machine increased, the revenue from vending machines and the profits that schools received were unaffected:** French, S. A., et al. 2001. *American Journal of Public Health* 91(1):112-117.

p. 197   Table: **Schools That Allow Food Promotion or Advertising:** Adapted from Wechsler, H., N. D. Brener, S. Juester, and C. Miller. 2001. *Journal of School Health* 71(7):313-324.

p. 198   **Kids' daily intake of carbonated drink consumption rises sharply at around the age of 8:** Rampersaud, G. C., et al. 2003. *Journal of the American Dietetic Association* 103:97-100.

p. 198   **Two-thirds of American adolescent girls and three-quarters of adolescent boys drink soft drinks daily:** Borrud, L., et al. 1997. What we eat: USDA surveys food consumption changes. Community Nutrition Institute Newsletter. Pp. 4-5.

p. 198   **researchers found that the more soda or sugar-sweetened drinks kids drink each day, the greater their risk of becoming obese:** Ludwig, D. S., et al. 2001. *Lancet* 357:505-508.

p. 198   **School authorities also issued new guidelines that reduced the amount of fat allowed in school lunches:** "Junk Food Banned from Vending Machines." Reuters. June 26, 2003.

p. 198   **with some schools reporting a drop in revenues from vending machines when sodas disappeared:** Merl, J. "Students learn to dispense with sodas." Los Angeles Times. February 12, 2004.

p. 199   **In August, 2003 school district officials were considering an exclusivity contract with a soft drink company:** Snyder, S. "Views vary on school soda sales." Philadelphia Inquirer. August 27, 2003.

p. 199   **after widespread public criticism of the deal, they had re-
treated from the contract idea:** Hardy, D. "Schools wary of soda deals."
Philadelphia Inquirer. January 22, 2004.

p. 199   **At middle and junior high schools, sodas may not be sold during regular school hours:** Litz, P. "Soda sales fizzed out in local schools." Los
Angeles Times. September 19, 2003. California Senate Bill No. 677. Chapter
415.

p. 199   **schools would no longer be permitted to sell foods that compete with the cafeteria's official breakfast, lunch, and after-school snack
offerings:** Russell Hughes, P. "State orders schools to cut out junk food."
Houston Chronicle. March 4, 2004.

p. 199   **"Policymakers should try to increase the quantity and quality of physical education":** NSDA Statement on Efforts to Ban or Restrict
the Sale of Carbonated Beverages in Schools. National Soft Drink Association, August 27, 2002. [Online]. Available at: http://www.nsda.org/
pressroom/2002_statementonbans.asp [accessed November 12, 2004].

p. 200   **The company also announced that it would no longer offer
schools the large one-time payments:** Coca Cola Issues Model Guidelines
for School Beverage Partnerships. News release, The Coca-Cola Company,
November 17, 2003. [Online]. Available at: http://www2.coca-cola.com/
presscenter/nr_20031117_school_model_guidelines.html [accessed November, 12, 2004].

CHAPTER 8

p. 216   **(In children younger than 3 years old, being fat has been
found not to predict future obesity risk.):** Whitaker, R. C., et al. 1997. *New
England Journal of Medicine* 337:869-873.

p. 216   **In 1994 Epstein reported the results of 10 years of follow-up
among 158 children he had treated for obesity:** Epstein, L. H., et al. 1994.
Health Psychology 13(5):373-383.

p. 217   **"Successful behavioral programs are labor intensive":**
Yanovski, J. A., and S. Z. Yanovski. 2003. *JAMA* 289(14):1851-1853.

p. 219   **Most overweight children do not need to undergo a battery
of expensive laboratory tests:** Moran, R. 1999. *American Family Physician*
59(4):861-868.

p. 222   **The 2005 edition of the federal government's dietary guidelines:** United States Department of Agriculture. 2005. Report of the Dietary
Guidelines Advisory Committee on the Dietary Guidelines for Americans.
[Online]. Available at: http://www.health.gov/dietaryguidelines/dga2005/
report [accessed November 12, 2004].

p. 222   **The Stoplight Diet . . . is another approach to changing children's eating habits:** Epstein, L. H., and S. S. Squires. 1988. *The Stoplight Diet for Children.* Boston: Little, Brown and Co.

p. 225   **Current guidelines for doctors treating overweight kids advise:** Barlow, S. E., and W. H. Dietz. 1998. *Pediatrics* 102(3):e29.

p. 229   **The only published scientific trial of its effectiveness was done in adolescents between the ages of 12 and 18:** Mellin, L. M., et al. 1987. *Journal of the American Dietetic Association.* 87(3):333-338.

p. 230   **A program using a similar approach, without the physical activity component:** Figueroa-Colon, R., et al. 1993. *American Journal of Diseases of Children* 147:160-166; Figueroa-Colon, R., et al. 1996. *Obesity Research* 4:419-429.

p. 230   **(However, the results in the 37 adolescents who declined to be evaluated may have been quite different.):** Sothern, M. S., et al. 2002. *Journal of the American Dietetic Association* 102:S81-S85.

p. 232   **Orlistat has recently been approved for obese children 12 years old or older:** Food and Drug Administration. NDA 20-766/S-018. [Online]. Available at: http://www.fda.gov/medwatch/SAFETY/2003/ 03DEC_PI/Xenical_PI.pdf [accessed November 12, 2004].

p. 232   **However, a large number of participants dropped out of both groups:** James, W. P., et al. 2000. *Lancet* 356:2119-2125.

p. 232   **Robert Berkowitz conducted a trial of sibutramine in overweight teenagers:** Berkowitz, R. I., et al. 2003. *JAMA* 289:1805-1812.

p. 233   **The best evidence supporting metformin's value in delaying diabetes comes from the Diabetes Prevention Program:** Knowler, W. C., et al. 2002. *New England Journal of Medicine* 346:393-403.

pp. 233-234   **"Through its ability to reduce fasting blood glucose and insulin concentrations and to moderate weight gain":** Freemark, M., and D. Bursey. 2001. *Pediatrics* 107:E55.

p. 234   **"the National Institutes of Health guidelines state that herbal preparations are not recommended as part of a weight-loss program":** Yanovski, S. Z., and J. A. Yanovski. 2002. *New England Journal of Medicine* 346:591-602.

p. 241   **The annual chance of dying was 4.5 percent in patients who had not had the surgery:** MacDonald, K. G., et al. 1997. *Journal of Gastrointestinal Surgery* 1:213-220.

p. 242   **Most patients lost weight successfully and kept off significant amounts:** Sugerman, H. J., et al. 2003. *Journal of Gastrointestinal Surgery* Jan;7(1):102-107.

p. 242   **These deaths occurred 15 months and 3 $^1/_2$ years, respectively, after the procedure:** Breaux, C. W. 1995. *Obesity Surgery* 5:279-284.

p. 242   **Surgeons and obesity experts at Cincinnati Children's Hospital Medical Center have proposed a carefully considered set of guidelines:** Inge, T. H., et al. 2004. *Pediatrics* 114:217-223.

p. 244   **"the durability of surgically induced weight loss among adolescents remains to be clearly defined":** Inge, T. H., op cit.

CHAPTER 9

p. 248   **"All flourish when people eat more, and all employ armies of lobbyists to discourage governments from doing anything to inhibit overeating":** Nestle, M. 2003. *Science* 299:781.

p. 248   **"Very little is happening at the top. A lot is happening at the bottom":** "The Obesigenic Environment and How to Deal With It," an address by Kelly D. Brownell, presented at a symposium entitled Downsizing America: The Obesity Epidemic. Monday April 12, 2004.

p. 251   **food and beverage advertisers currently spend between $10 billion and $12 billion each year to reach children and youth:** Brownell, K. D., and K. B. Horgen. 2004. *Food Fight: The Inside Story of the Food Industry, America's Obesity Crisis and What We Can Do About It.* New York: McGraw-Hill; Nestle, M. J. 2002. *Food Politics: How the Food Industry Influences Nutrition and Health.* Berkeley, CA: University of California Press.

p. 251   **In 2002 annual sales of foods and drinks to children and adolescents in the United States totaled more than $27 billion:** U.S. Market for Kids Foods and Beverages. June 2003. Fifth Edition. [Online]. Available at: http://www.marketresearch.com/rcsearchindex/849192.html#pagetop [accessed November 12, 2004].

p. 251   **concluded that "more than 50 percent of television advertisements directed at children promote foods and beverages such a candy, fast food":** Koplan, J. P., et al., eds. 2005. *Preventing Childhood Obesity: Health in the Balance.* Institute of Medicine. Washington, DC: The National Academies Press.

p. 251   **Children see one food commercial, on average, during every five minutes of television that they watch:** Kotz, K., and M. Story. 1994. *Journal of the American Dietetic Association* 94:1296-1300.

p. 251   **Channel One . . . reaches an estimated eight million teenage students in more than 350,000 classrooms . . . shows 10 minutes of news and 2 minutes of commercials each day:** Primedia Inc., Channel One network. [Online]. Available at: http://www.primediainc.com [accessed November 12, 2004].

p. 252   **researchers found that more than two-thirds of Channel One's commercials were for food products:** Brand, J., and B. Greenberg. 1994. *Journal of Advertising Research* 34:18-23.

p. 252   Candy, cereal, and pizza makers also offer schools free "educational materials" featuring math or science lessons that use their products: Brownell, K. D., and K. B. Horgen, op cit.

p. 252   Advertising's specific impact on children's diet has been difficult to quantify because so many factors influence food choices: Hastings, G., et al. 2003. *Review of Research on the Effects of Food Promotion to Children.* Glasgow, UK: Center for Social Marketing, University of Strathclyde.

p. 252   "Wider impacts include the increased consumption of energy-dense foods and beverages and greater engagement in sedentary behaviors": Koplan, J. P., et al., op cit.

p. 252   before the age of about 7 or 8, they don't even understand that the purpose of an advertisement is to persuade, rather than to entertain or to inform: Wilcox, B. L., et al. 2004. *Report of the APA Task Force on Advertising and Children.* Washington, DC: American Psychological Association.

p. 252   the American Academy of Pediatrics in 1995 issued a policy statement that "advertising directed toward children is inherently deceptive and exploits children under 8 years of age": American Academy of Pediatrics, Committee on Communications. 1995. *Pediatrics* 95(2):295-297.

p. 252   61 percent of respondents agreed with the statement that "advertising to children begins at too young an age": Harris Interactive. Youth Marketers Feel It Is Appropriate to Begin Marketing to Kids at Age Seven. [Online]. Available at: http://www.harrisinteractive.com/news/allnewsbydate.asp?NewsID=792 [accessed on November 12, 2004].

p. 253   to restrict television advertising to children, on the grounds that all advertising that is directed at children too young to understand an ad's intent is inherently unfair and deceptive: In the Matter of Children's Advertising. 1978. 43 Fed. Reg. 17967.

p. 253   Congress passed a law in 1980 withdrawing the FTC's authority to restrict children's advertising and prohibiting it from adopting the proposed rules: Federal Trade Commission Improvements Act of 1980. PL 96-252.

p. 253   A renewed effort by the FTC to limit advertising to children would likely suffer from the same drawbacks as the 1970s effort: Engle, M. K. 2003. FTC Regulation of Marketing to Children. Presentation at the workshop on the Prevention of Childhood Obesity: Understanding the Influences of Marketing, Media and Family Dynamics. Committee on the Prevention of Obesity in Children and Youth, Institute of Medicine, Washington, DC. December 9, 2003.

p. 253   "As an industry, we strongly reject the claims that advertising causes childhood obesity": Pereira, J., and A. Warren. Wall Street Journal. March 15, 2004. B1.

pp. 254-255   **Parents should find out whether Channel One and other sources of advertising are present in their local schools:** Koplan, J. P., et al., op cit.

p. 255   **He cited the association's successful suit several years ago by state attorneys general against tobacco companies:** Reeves, A. *Investor's Business Daily.* June 21, 2004. [Online]. Available at: http://www.investors.com.

p. 256   **People who live in mixed-use neighborhoods with access to shops and public transportation tend to walk more, and to weigh less:** Frank, L. D., et al. 2004. *American Journal of Preventive Medicine* 27:87-96.

p. 257   **the percentage of children walking or biking to school increased from 21 percent when the program started to 38 percent two years later:** Miller, L. Communities hoping to get kids walking to school again. Associated Press. June 23, 2003.

p. 257   **If local residents educate themselves about zoning and school district policies, they can become advocates for the preservation of existing schools:** Historic Neighborhood Schools in the Age of Sprawl: Why Johnny Can't Walk to School. 2000. The National Trust for Historic Preservation.

p. 261   **A similar although smaller dose-response effect of supermarkets on fruit and vegetable intake:** Morland, K., et al. 2002. *American Journal of Public Health* 92(11):1761-1767.

p. 261   **the Food Trust ... mapped the locations of supermarket sales within the city and compared them with a map of mortality rates from diet-related diseases:** The Food Trust. 2001. "Food for Every Child." [Online]. Available at: http://www.thefoodtrust.org [accessed November, 12, 2004].

p. 263   **The number of farmers markets in the United States increased by more than 75 percent:** United States Department of Agriculture. [Online]. Available at: http://www.ams.usda.gov/farmersmarkets/ FarmersMarket Growth.htm [accessed November 12, 2004].

Acknowledgments

F *ed Up!* would not have been possible without the generous support of the Institute of Medicine (IOM) and the Robert Wood Johnson Foundation. I am also grateful to many individuals for their assistance and encouragement during the research and writing of this book. First, my thanks to Harvey Fineberg and Mary Wilson, beloved friends and mentors, for suggesting that I write a book for the general audience on this topic. I also thank the members of the IOM Committee on Prevention of Obesity in Children and Youth, as well as Cathy Liverman, Linda Meyers, and their wonderful staff. Special thanks to Vivica Kraak, Shannon Ruddy Wisham, and Janice Okita for putting up with my pestering.

On the IOM committee, Shiriki Kumanyika helped guide my reporting and generously read and commented on the entire manuscript; Jeffrey Koplan, Russell Pate, Robert Whitaker, Leann Birch, and Dennis Bier offered valuable feedback on various chapters. I am also indebted to Tom Robinson, Douglas Kamerow, Leann Birch, and Susan Handy for interviews and other assistance during my research. The committee's report, *Preventing Childhood Obesity: Health in the Balance,* was an essential resource during the later stages of my writing.

I especially thank Rudy Leibel for tutoring me in the genetics and physiology of body weight regulation, answering countless questions via e-mail, and suggesting changes that immeasurably improved Chapter 2. Others who helped me learn about the biology of appetite and obesity were Michael Schwartz, David Cummings, Matthias Tschöp, Eric Ravussin, Antonio Tataranni, Robert Nelson, Albert J. Stunkard, and Nicolas Stettler. Julie Mennella taught me about the development of taste and smell in the fetus and infant.

At the National Institutes of Health, Jack Yanovski introduced me to the epidemiology and treatment of pediatric obesity and Philip Smith provided an overview of obesity research. Sue Yanovski and Deborah Young-Hyman helped with my reporting and offered important feedback on the chapters about self-esteem and obesity treatment. Robert Kuczmarski kindly shared his personal and family strategies for building physical activity into daily life.

Special thanks to Bill Dietz and Steve Gortmaker for making available their broad knowledge of childhood nutrition and obesity prevention. The work of Robert Whitaker and Simone French deepened my understanding of environmental influences on food intake and energy balance. At the Centers for Disease Control, my thanks to Venkat Narayan for information on rising rates of diabetes and to Katherine Flegal for explaining the epidemic's impact on the distribution of BMIs in the population. At the U.S. Department of Agriculture, Suanne Buggy of the Food and Nutrition Service answered my questions about the federal school lunch program.

For help in understanding the psychological impact of obesity on children and adolescents, I am indebted to Michael Rich of Children's Hospital Boston, to the research of Marla Eisenberg and Deborah Young-Hyman, and to Minda Barnett, Atalaya Sergi, Tracey Saxon, Joyce Green Pastors, and the girls of the Bold and Beautiful Club in Charlottesville. For giving me a close-up look at how kids live today, I especially thank Meagan, her family and friends, and the teachers and administrators at her school (which I do not name for reasons of privacy); Brian and his mother, Cassandra; English teacher Ray Devenney and his students at Washington, D.C.'s Bell Multicultural High School; my own students at Georgetown Day School; and Christine Mattis, John Hankey, and the students at D. W. Griffith Junior High School in East Los Angeles.

Nazrat Mirza, Larry D'Angelo, and Terry Kind of Children's National Medical Center in Washington, D.C., Leonard Epstein in Buffalo, Nancy McLaren in Charlottesville, and Robert I. Berkowitz and Thomas A. Wadden of the University of Pennsylvania shared their expertise on obesity treatment. Daniel Davidow and Anne C. Leary of Virginia's Cumberland Hospital provided insight into the sobering challenge of treating extreme obesity in children and adolescents. In Charlottesville, Milagros Huerta and Erika Zeff of the University of Virginia Health System allowed me to visit a pediatric obesity treatment program that has been integrated with a primary care system. Surgeons H. David Reines, Thomas Inge, Victor Garcia, Walter Pories, and Harvey Sugerman taught me about bariatric surgery and illuminated the debate over its use in adolescents. Thanks also to Melinda Sothern of Committed to Kids, Bob Mellin of Shapedown, Chris Corcoran of WeightWatchers, and Cathy Garvey of Jenny Craig for information on their programs and to dietitian Susan Baum of INOVA Fairfax Hospital.

For imparting their knowledge of healthy ways of eating, I am grateful to David L. Katz, David Ludwig, Walter C. Willett, and Leonard Epstein. Marion Nestle, Maureen Black, and Margaret Bentley helped me find answers to specific nutrition questions. The work of Barbara Rolls, Leann Birch, Jennifer Fisher, and Jane Wardle taught me much about how the environment influences children's food intake and preferences. Vivica Kraak and the IOM committee staff provided especially valuable guidance on Chapter 4. Adam, Bruce, Trianna, and their parents proved to me that kids and families can indeed transform their eating habits. Sheila Crye shared insights from teaching cooking classes to children. Esther Cook, Amanda Rieux, and the staff and students of the Edible Schoolyard program at Berkeley's Martin Luther King Middle School hosted me for an idyllic morning in their garden and kitchen.

In Kansas City, many thanks to Joseph Donnelly, Janet May, and staff members of the University of Kansas PAAC program and to the teachers and students at Briarwood Elementary, Prairie Elementary, and Brookridge Elementary in the Shawnee Mission School District. The work of Tom Robinson, Steve Gortmaker, and Michael Goran especially helped me understand how children's activity levels and leisure habits influence obesity rates. I am grateful to James Sallis of San Diego State University and to James Hill of the University of Colorado for discussing strategies for increasing physical activity.

Obstetricians Frank Witter and Joan Loveland lent their expertise to the section on pregnancy, and the work of Matthew Gillman, David Barker, and Michael Kramer taught me about prenatal contributors to children's future obesity risk. Lactation consultant Debbie Tobin of INOVA Fairfax Hospital allowed me to attend her breastfeeding support group and helped me locate resources. My thanks to Linda, Kristen, and their daughters. Barbara Moore's workshop on environmental influences during pregnancy, infancy, and early childhood proved invaluable.

In Boston, Jill Carter, Stacy Johnson, and Lillian Cheung arranged for me to visit public schools to observe teachers using innovative curricula on nutrition and physical activity. I am especially grateful to principals Shirley Allen of Mildred Avenue Middle School, Deborah Dancy of Channing Elementary, and Suzanne Lee of Josiah Quincy School and to their faculty and students. Epidemiologist Leslie Lytle helped me interpret the CATCH program's results. Meg Campbell shared the philosophy behind her unique "walking school" at Codman Academy.

At the Food Trust in Philadelphia, Megan McGreevy, Sandy Sherman, Karima Rose, Dan Lewis, Brian Lang, and Hannah Burton shared their organization's inventive strategies for improving the nutrition of children and adults in their community. My thanks to the children and teachers involved in the student-run fruit stand project at North Philadelphia's Fairhill Elementary.

The legislative and policy issues surrounding nutrition, obesity, and physical activity can be overwhelming without a road map. For help with navigation, I am grateful to Linda Meyers of the National

Academies, Susan Foerster of the California Department of Health Services, Kim Stitzel and Jessica Donze of the American Dietetic Association, and Leslie Mikkelsen of the Prevention Institute in Oakland, California. My thanks to Lisa Kelly and Parker Lawton of the International Food Information Council Foundation for compiling an invaluable digest of media coverage of obesity. Mary K. Engle of the Federal Trade Commission reviewed the section on her agency's past efforts to regulate advertising to children, and Susan Linn and Vivica Kraak provided information on current marketing practices. Marion Nestle, Kelly Brownell, Adam Drewnowski, and Roland Sturm gave me a deeper understanding of how economic and political factors influence obesity prevalence as well as prevention and treatment. Joel Gittelsohn introduced me to the Healthy Stores Project.

I especially thank Nancy McLaren and Phil Nieburg for helping me learn how members of one community—Charlottesville—have come together to fight childhood obesity. Peggy Paviour and Barbara Yager of the Thomas Jefferson Health District of the Virginia Department of Health inspired me with their success in documenting the epidemic in Charlottesville and mobilizing leaders and community residents to respond.

My thanks to Tom Wilkinson and Liz Spayd of the *Washington Post* for allowing me professional leave to write this book, to Rich Chefetz for urging me to take the leap, and to my journalistic colleagues Curt Suplee, Kathy Sawyer, Sally Squires, Rick Weiss, David Brown, Sandy Boodman, Dale Russakoff, Rob Stein, and Madeline Drexler for assistance and advice.

I am grateful for the enthusiasm and professionalism of Stephen Mautner and his colleagues at the Joseph Henry Press, including the design, production, and marketing staff for their stellar work. Above all, I thank my wonderful editor, Mary Kalamaras, for her support, her insightful feedback, her meticulous editing, and her passionate dedication to this project. My thanks to Chris Jerome for her graceful copy editing.

Finally, I thank my husband, Walter Weiss, my sons Peter and Jacob, and my brother Rick Okie for their love and encouragement during the two years I spent researching and writing *Fed Up!*

Index

C